This publication is intended to provide educational information for the reader on the covered subjects. It is not intended to take the place of personalized medical counseling, diagnosis, and treatment from a trained healthcare professional.

ISBN 978-1-998455-89-8 (Paperback)
ISBN 978-1-998455-90-4 (eBook)

Printed and bound in USA
Published by Loons Press

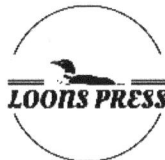

LOONS PRESS

# Table Of Contents

# How To Reduce Esophageal Cancer Risk

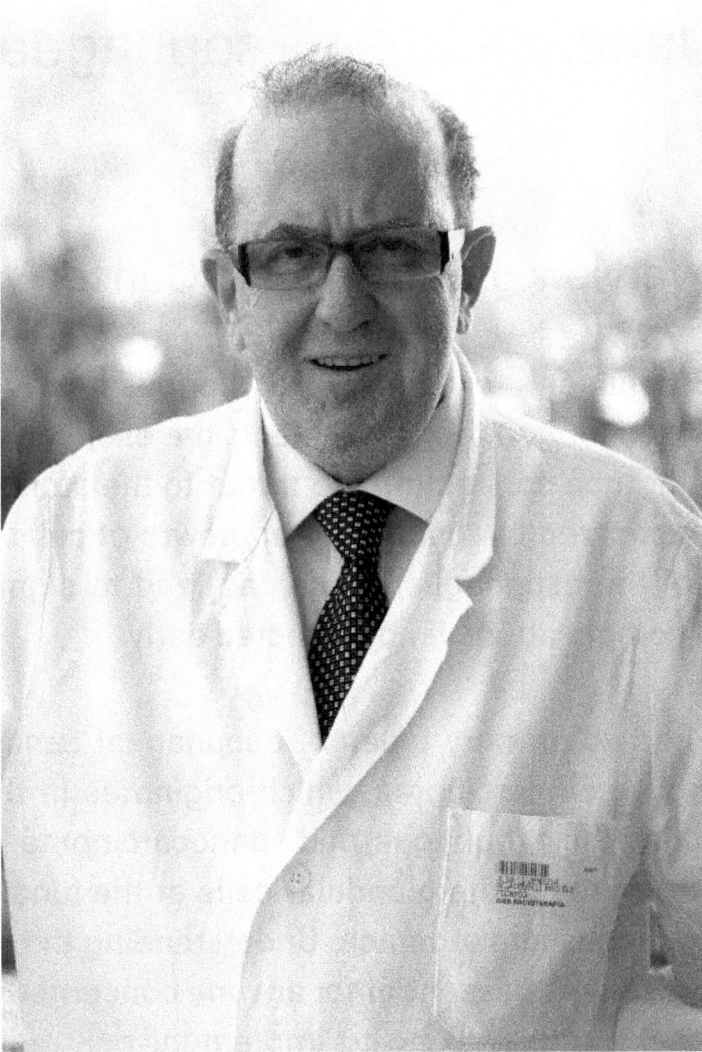

A Comprehensive Guide

# Chapter 1

# Understanding Esophageal Cancer

## Overview of Esophageal Cancer

Esophageal cancer is a serious and often overlooked malignancy that affects the esophagus, the muscular tube connecting the throat to the stomach. It is characterized by the abnormal growth of cells in the lining of the esophagus, which can lead to significant health complications if not detected early.

The two primary types of esophageal cancer are squamous cell carcinoma, which originates in the flat cells lining the esophagus, and adenocarcinoma, which typically arises in the glandular cells at the junction of the esophagus and stomach. Understanding the nature of this disease is essential for anyone concerned about their health and seeking to implement risk reduction strategies.

The incidence of esophageal cancer has been rising in recent decades, particularly in Western countries. Risk factors are diverse and can include lifestyle choices, environmental influences, and underlying health conditions. Tobacco use, excessive alcohol consumption, obesity, and chronic gastroesophageal reflux disease (GERD) are among the most significant contributors to the development of this disease.

Additionally, certain dietary habits, such as low intake of fruits and vegetables, and exposure to specific chemicals or irritants can further elevate the risk. By identifying these risk factors, individuals can take proactive steps to mitigate their chances of developing esophageal cancer.

Symptoms of esophageal cancer often do not manifest until the disease is in advanced stages, making early detection challenging. Common signs include difficulty swallowing, unintentional weight loss, persistent heartburn, and chest pain.

Due to the nonspecific nature of these symptoms, they can be mistaken for less serious conditions, which is why regular medical check-ups and awareness of personal risk factors are critical. Individuals who experience any of these symptoms should consult a healthcare professional promptly to rule out esophageal cancer or other serious health issues.

Preventive measures play a crucial role in reducing the risk of esophageal cancer. Lifestyle modifications such as quitting smoking, limiting alcohol intake, maintaining a healthy weight, and adopting a balanced diet rich in fruits and vegetables can significantly diminish the likelihood of developing this disease.

Additionally, managing acid reflux through dietary changes and medications can help alleviate chronic irritation of the esophagus, further decreasing cancer risk. Engaging in regular physical activity also contributes to overall health and can help maintain a healthy weight, which is a key factor in prevention.

In conclusion, an overview of esophageal cancer underscores the importance of awareness, early detection, and lifestyle modification. Individuals concerned about their risk should educate themselves on the disease's risk factors and symptoms, actively participate in preventive measures, and seek regular medical evaluations.

By understanding the nature of esophageal cancer and applying practical strategies for risk reduction, individuals can empower themselves to lead healthier lives and significantly decrease their chances of developing this serious condition.

## Risk Factors and Statistics

Esophageal cancer remains a significant health concern globally, with various risk factors contributing to its development. Understanding these risk factors is crucial for individuals seeking to minimize their chances of developing this disease. The primary risk factors include lifestyle choices such as smoking and excessive alcohol consumption, along with underlying health conditions like gastroesophageal reflux disease (GERD) and Barrett's esophagus.

Research indicates that smoking increases the risk of esophageal cancer by as much as 50%, while heavy alcohol consumption can exacerbate the effects of other risk factors.

Statistics play a vital role in understanding the prevalence and impact of esophageal cancer. According to the American Cancer Society, esophageal cancer is projected to account for approximately 20,640 new cases in the United States in a given year, with an estimated 15,620 deaths. The incidence of this cancer type has been on the rise, particularly among men and older adults.

Additionally, certain demographic factors, such as age, gender, and ethnicity, significantly influence risk levels. For instance, men are three to four times more likely to develop esophageal cancer than women, and rates are notably higher among individuals of Caucasian descent compared to African Americans and Hispanics.

Obesity is another critical risk factor linked to esophageal cancer, particularly the adenocarcinoma subtype. The correlation between obesity and GERD is well-documented; excess body weight increases abdominal pressure, which can lead to acid reflux and subsequent esophageal irritation.

Studies have shown that individuals with a body mass index (BMI) of 30 or higher are at an increased risk, making weight management an essential strategy for those concerned about esophageal cancer. Understanding the interplay between obesity, GERD, and cancer risk can empower individuals to adopt healthier lifestyles.

Diet also plays a crucial role in shaping risk factors associated with esophageal cancer. Diets high in processed meats, refined carbohydrates, and low in fruits and vegetables may elevate risk levels. Conversely, a diet rich in whole foods, particularly those high in antioxidants and fiber, has been associated with a reduced risk of esophageal cancer.

Nutritional strategies, such as incorporating more fruits, vegetables, and whole grains while reducing the intake of red and processed meats, can be effective in mitigating risk. Awareness of dietary influences can guide individuals toward healthier eating habits.

Finally, genetics and family history can further complicate risk factors for esophageal cancer. Individuals with a family history of this cancer or related conditions may face a higher risk due to inherited genetic predispositions. Genetic counseling can provide valuable insights for those concerned about their risk based on family history.

By combining knowledge of personal risk factors with proactive lifestyle changes, individuals can take significant steps toward reducing their likelihood of developing esophageal cancer, thus enhancing their overall health and well-being.

## Symptoms and Early Detection

Esophageal cancer often develops silently, which makes early detection crucial for effective treatment and improved outcomes. Understanding the symptoms that may indicate the presence of esophageal cancer is essential for individuals concerned about their health. Common symptoms include difficulty swallowing (dysphagia), persistent heartburn or gastroesophageal reflux disease (GERD), unintentional weight loss, and chest pain.

These symptoms can sometimes be mistaken for less serious conditions, which underscores the importance of consulting a healthcare provider if they persist. Being vigilant about changes in the body and seeking medical advice can lead to earlier diagnosis and better management of potential health issues.

Dysphagia, or difficulty swallowing, is often one of the first noticeable symptoms. Individuals may experience a sensation of food getting stuck in the throat or chest, leading to discomfort and anxiety during meals.

This symptom is particularly concerning because it can significantly impact dietary habits and nutritional intake. Alongside dysphagia, chronic heartburn or GERD can also signal esophageal irritation that, if left unchecked, could lead to more severe complications, including the development of Barrett's esophagus, a precursor to esophageal cancer. Recognizing these symptoms and understanding their potential implications is vital for anyone concerned about their risk.

Weight loss that occurs without trying is another alarming symptom that warrants immediate attention. In cases where the body struggles to intake food due to esophageal issues, individuals may unintentionally lose weight, which can lead to malnutrition and further health complications. Chest pain, often described as a burning sensation or discomfort, can also be symptomatic of esophageal cancer.

Though many may attribute these symptoms to anxiety or gastrointestinal disorders, persistent or worsening symptoms should never be ignored. Early medical evaluation can help differentiate between benign conditions and more serious concerns.

Regular screenings and checkups play a fundamental role in early detection, especially for individuals with known risk factors such as a history of smoking, excessive alcohol consumption, or chronic GERD. Healthcare providers may recommend endoscopic examinations or imaging tests for those showing symptoms or who are at higher risk. These proactive measures can lead to the identification of abnormal cells or lesions before they progress to cancer. Individuals should advocate for themselves by discussing their concerns with healthcare professionals and ensuring that they receive appropriate assessments based on their risk profile.

In summary, being informed about the symptoms and taking proactive steps towards early detection can significantly influence the outcomes of esophageal health. Individuals concerned about esophageal cancer should maintain open communication with their healthcare providers, prioritize regular screenings, and remain vigilant about any changes in their body. By recognizing the signs and seeking timely medical intervention, individuals can empower themselves to take control of their health and reduce their risk of esophageal cancer.

# How To Reduce Esophageal Cancer Risk

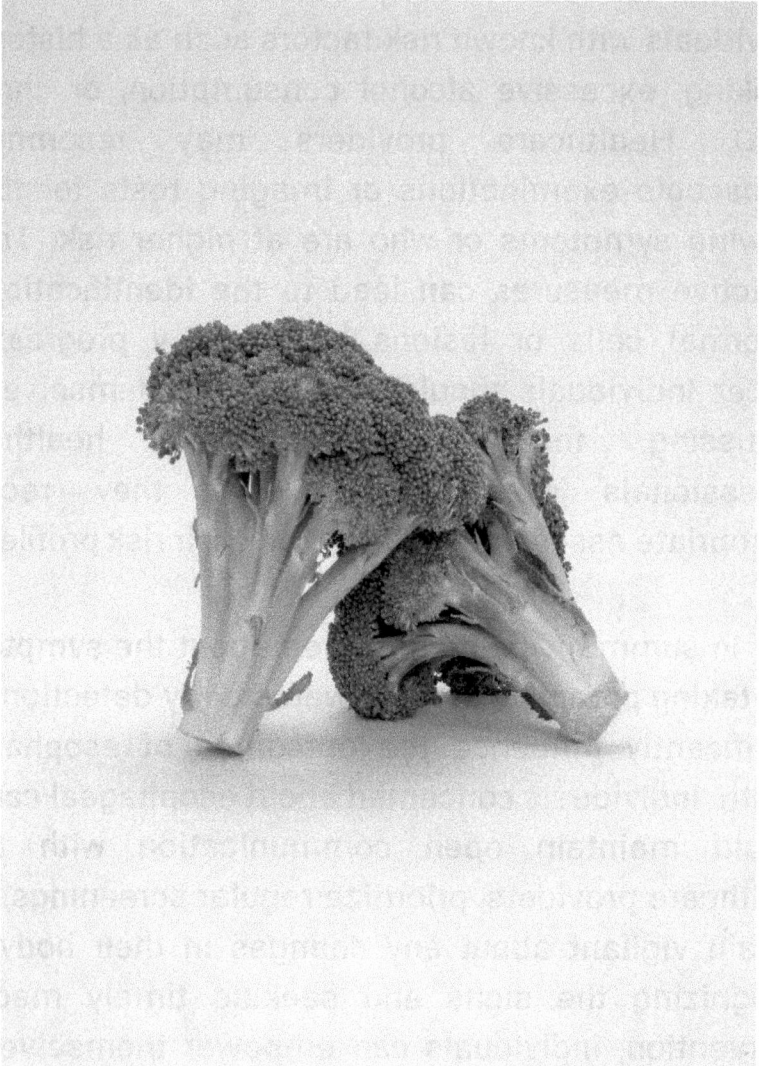

# Chapter 2

# The Role of Diet in Prevention

## Foods to Include for Esophageal Health

Esophageal health is a crucial aspect of overall well-being, particularly for individuals concerned about the risk of esophageal cancer. Incorporating specific foods into your diet can play a significant role in reducing this risk. This subchapter examines the various food categories that promote esophageal health, emphasizing nutrient-dense options that support the body's natural defenses against cancer.

Fruits and vegetables are at the forefront of a diet designed to enhance esophageal health. Rich in vitamins, minerals, and antioxidants, these foods help combat oxidative stress and inflammation, both of which are linked to cancer development.

Cruciferous vegetables, such as broccoli, cauliflower, and Brussels sprouts, contain compounds like sulforaphane that have been shown to have anti-cancer properties. Including a variety of colorful fruits, such as berries, citrus, and dark leafy greens, ensures a broad spectrum of phytonutrients, which can help bolster the immune system and promote cellular health.

Whole grains should also be emphasized in a diet aimed at reducing esophageal cancer risk. Foods such as brown rice, quinoa, whole wheat bread, and oats provide essential fiber, which supports digestive health and can help maintain a healthy weight.

High-fiber diets are associated with a lower risk of various cancers, including those of the digestive tract. Additionally, whole grains are rich in B vitamins and minerals like magnesium and selenium, which contribute to overall health and may help protect against cancerous changes in cells.

Protein sources should be selected with care, as they can influence esophageal health. Lean proteins, such as fish, skinless poultry, legumes, and low-fat dairy, are beneficial options. Fatty fish like salmon and mackerel are particularly valuable due to their high omega-3 fatty acid content, which has been shown to have anti-inflammatory properties.

Reducing consumption of processed meats and high-fat red meats is recommended, as these have been linked to an increased risk of various cancers, including esophageal cancer.

Finally, healthy fats play a vital role in a balanced diet. Incorporating sources of monounsaturated and polyunsaturated fats, such as olive oil, avocados, nuts, and seeds, can support cellular health and reduce inflammation. These fats not only contribute to heart health but also aid in the absorption of fat-soluble vitamins, which are essential for maintaining overall health. It is advisable to limit trans fats and saturated fats found in fried and processed foods, as these can exacerbate inflammation and negatively impact overall health.

In summary, focusing on a diet rich in fruits, vegetables, whole grains, lean proteins, and healthy fats can significantly contribute to esophageal health and reduce the risk of esophageal cancer. By making informed dietary choices and prioritizing nutrient-dense foods, individuals can empower themselves in the fight against cancer, promoting not only esophageal well-being but also enhancing their overall health.

## Foods to Avoid

In the quest to reduce the risk of esophageal cancer, understanding dietary choices plays a crucial role. Certain foods have been associated with an increased likelihood of developing this type of cancer, and avoiding them can be a proactive step towards better health.

This subchapter focuses on specific foods and food groups that individuals concerned about esophageal cancer should consider eliminating or significantly reducing from their diets.

Processed meats are among the most critical foods to avoid. Studies have shown a strong correlation between the consumption of processed meats—such as sausages, bacon, and deli meats—and an elevated risk of esophageal cancer. These products often contain preservatives like nitrates and nitrites, which can form carcinogenic compounds when cooked at high temperatures. Reducing or eliminating processed meats from your diet can significantly lower cancer risk while also improving overall health.

High-temperature cooking methods, such as grilling and frying, can create harmful compounds in foods. For instance, charred or burnt foods contain polycyclic aromatic hydrocarbons (PAHs) and advanced glycation end products (AGEs), both of which have been linked to an increased risk of cancer. Individuals should be mindful of the cooking techniques they use and consider healthier options like steaming, boiling, or baking to minimize exposure to these harmful substances. Additionally, it is advisable to avoid heavily charred or burnt foods, as they may contribute to inflammation and cellular damage.

Another category of foods to avoid includes those high in refined sugars and carbohydrates. Diets laden with sugary snacks, sodas, and white bread can lead to obesity, which is a significant risk factor for esophageal cancer. Excess body weight can increase the likelihood of gastroesophageal reflux disease (GERD), a condition that can further elevate cancer risk. Opting for whole grains, fruits, and vegetables instead can help maintain a healthy weight and provide essential nutrients that support overall well-being.

Acidic foods and beverages, particularly those high in citric acid, can exacerbate GERD symptoms, increasing the risk of esophageal cancer over time. Citrus fruits, vinegar, and certain carbonated drinks are known to contribute to acid reflux.

While these foods can be enjoyed in moderation by individuals without GERD, those concerned about esophageal cancer should limit their intake and monitor their body's response. Substituting with less acidic options, like non-citrus fruits and herbal teas, can provide flavor and enjoyment without the added risk.

In conclusion, making informed dietary choices is a significant step towards reducing the risk of esophageal cancer. By avoiding processed meats, high-temperature cooked foods, refined sugars, and acidic items, individuals can create a healthier eating pattern that supports their overall health and lowers cancer risk.

These practical strategies not only serve as a preventive measure but also contribute to a more balanced and nutritious diet, fostering long-term wellness.

## The Importance of Hydration

Hydration plays a crucial role in maintaining overall health and well-being, and its significance extends to the prevention of esophageal cancer. Proper hydration helps the body function optimally, allowing for efficient digestion and nutrient absorption.

The esophagus, being a critical component of the digestive system, benefits from adequate fluid intake. When the body is well-hydrated, the esophagus is better protected against irritation and damage that may contribute to cancer development. Thus, understanding the importance of hydration is essential for individuals concerned about their risk of esophageal cancer.

Water serves as a natural lubricant for the entire digestive tract, facilitating the smooth passage of food from the mouth to the stomach. Insufficient hydration can lead to dry mouth and difficulty swallowing, increasing the likelihood of food particles becoming lodged in the esophagus.

Chronic irritation from these particles can cause inflammation, which is a known risk factor for esophageal cancer. By ensuring proper hydration, individuals can support healthy swallowing and reduce the risk of mechanical damage to the esophagus.

Moreover, hydration is vital for maintaining the mucosal lining of the esophagus. This lining acts as a barrier protecting the esophagus from harmful substances, including acidic contents from the stomach. When dehydrated, the mucosal barrier may weaken, making the esophagus more susceptible to injury from acid reflux and other irritants.

Chronic acid exposure is a significant risk factor for conditions like Barrett's esophagus, which can lead to esophageal cancer. Therefore, staying adequately hydrated can help preserve the integrity of the esophageal lining and minimize the risk of such damaging conditions.

The quality of the fluids consumed is also important in the context of esophageal cancer prevention. While water is the best choice for hydration, other beverages can play a role as well. However, individuals should be cautious with drinks that are highly acidic, caffeinated, or alcoholic, as these can irritate the esophagus and exacerbate reflux symptoms.

Instead, incorporating herbal teas, non-citrus juices, and infused waters can provide hydration without the associated risks of more harmful beverages. Developing a habit of choosing hydrating, non-irritating drinks can significantly contribute to long-term esophageal health.

In conclusion, adequate hydration is a fundamental yet often overlooked strategy for reducing the risk of esophageal cancer. By promoting healthy digestion, supporting the mucosal lining, and making mindful choices about beverage consumption, individuals can take proactive steps toward protecting their esophagus.

Establishing a routine that prioritizes hydration not only fosters overall health but also serves as a practical measure in the broader context of esophageal cancer prevention. As individuals become more aware of the importance of hydration, they can empower themselves to make informed choices that contribute to their long-term well-being.

# How To Reduce Esophageal Cancer Risk

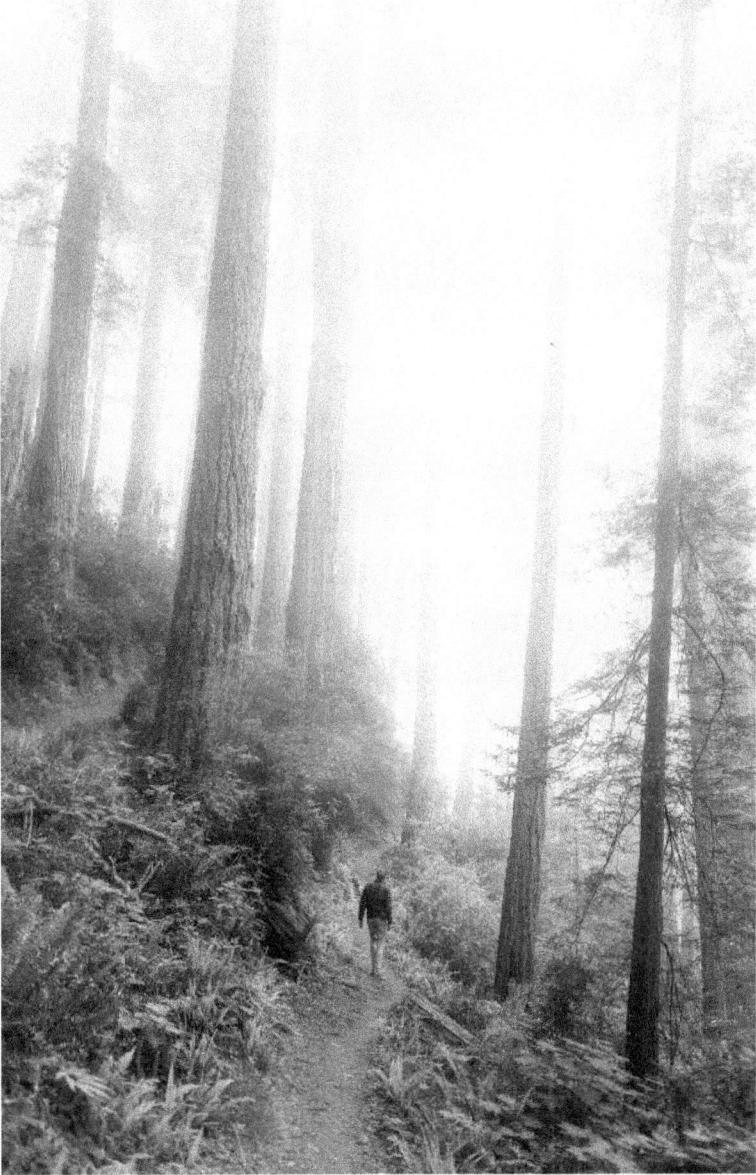

# Chapter 3

# Lifestyle Modifications

## Maintaining a Healthy Weight

Maintaining a healthy weight is a crucial aspect of reducing the risk of esophageal cancer. Research indicates a strong correlation between obesity and the incidence of this type of cancer, particularly esophageal adenocarcinoma. Excess body weight can lead to various metabolic changes, including increased inflammation and altered hormone levels, which may contribute to the development of cancer.

For individuals concerned about esophageal cancer, understanding the importance of weight management is essential for implementing effective risk reduction strategies.

A balanced diet plays a pivotal role in maintaining a healthy weight. Emphasizing whole foods such as fruits, vegetables, whole grains, lean proteins, and healthy fats can help individuals achieve and sustain an optimal weight. These foods are not only nutrient-dense but also lower in calories compared to processed and high-sugar options.

A focus on portion control and mindful eating can further support weight management efforts. It is beneficial to plan meals that prioritize these nutritious foods while minimizing the intake of high-calorie, low-nutrient items, such as sugary snacks and fast food.

In addition to dietary changes, regular physical activity is vital for weight maintenance. Engaging in moderate-intensity exercise, such as brisk walking, cycling, or swimming, for at least 150 minutes a week can greatly assist in achieving and sustaining a healthy weight. Incorporating strength training exercises at least twice a week can also boost metabolism and enhance muscle mass, which is important for long-term weight management.

For those who may be new to exercise, starting with small, manageable goals and gradually increasing intensity and duration can lead to sustainable habits.

Behavioral strategies can further support weight management efforts. Keeping a food diary, for instance, can increase awareness of eating habits and identify areas for improvement. Setting realistic and achievable weight loss or maintenance goals can also provide motivation and accountability. Additionally, seeking support from friends, family, or weight loss groups can create a sense of community and encouragement, making the journey toward a healthier weight feel less daunting and more achievable.

Lastly, it is important to recognize that maintaining a healthy weight is not just about aesthetics; it is a significant factor in overall health and well-being. Individuals concerned about esophageal cancer should view weight management as a holistic approach that encompasses lifestyle changes, emotional health, and medical guidance when necessary.

Regular check-ups with healthcare professionals can provide personalized advice and track progress, ensuring that individuals remain on the right path toward reducing their risk of esophageal cancer through effective weight management strategies.

## The Impact of Physical Activity

The impact of physical activity on overall health is widely acknowledged, but its specific role in reducing the risk of esophageal cancer has garnered increasing attention in recent years. Regular physical activity contributes to maintaining a healthy weight, enhancing the immune system, and improving gastrointestinal health—all factors that can play a significant role in cancer prevention.

Engaging in consistent exercise not only helps in managing body weight but also promotes the efficient functioning of metabolic processes, which can reduce inflammation and the likelihood of developing conditions associated with cancer.

Research has shown that individuals who lead sedentary lifestyles are at a higher risk of developing various types of cancer, including esophageal cancer. Obesity, in particular, is a well-established risk factor linked to this disease. Excess body weight can lead to gastroesophageal reflux disease (GERD), a condition where stomach acid frequently flows back into the esophagus, increasing the likelihood of cellular changes that may lead to cancer.

By incorporating regular physical activity into daily routines, individuals can effectively manage their weight and mitigate the risk factors associated with obesity and GERD.

The type and intensity of physical activity also matter when considering their impact on esophageal cancer risk. Aerobic exercises, such as brisk walking, running, swimming, or cycling, have been shown to improve cardiovascular health and enhance overall physical endurance. Strength training, on the other hand, can aid in muscle preservation and improve metabolic efficiency.

A well-rounded exercise regimen that includes both aerobic and resistance training is ideal for optimizing health outcomes. This holistic approach not only fosters weight management but also improves the body's ability to combat inflammation and oxidative stress, both of which are implicated in cancer development.

Moreover, the psychological benefits of physical activity cannot be overlooked. Regular exercise has been associated with reduced stress, anxiety, and depression, which can contribute to healthier lifestyle choices. Individuals who engage in physical activity are often more motivated to make dietary changes, avoid harmful behaviors, and adhere to medical recommendations.

This interconnectedness suggests that by prioritizing physical activity, individuals can create a positive feedback loop that reinforces other risk-reducing behaviors related to esophageal cancer.

In conclusion, the impact of physical activity extends far beyond mere weight management; it plays a crucial role in reducing the risk of esophageal cancer through its effects on body weight, metabolic health, and psychological well-being. For individuals concerned about their esophageal cancer risk, cultivating a consistent exercise routine can serve as a practical strategy for prevention. By understanding and harnessing the benefits of physical activity, individuals can take proactive steps toward safeguarding their health and reducing their vulnerability to this serious disease.

## Smoking Cessation Strategies

Smoking is a well-established risk factor for esophageal cancer, particularly for squamous cell carcinoma. The harmful chemicals in tobacco not only damage the cells of the esophagus but also lead to chronic inflammation and changes in cellular structure over time. For individuals concerned about their risk of esophageal cancer, quitting smoking is one of the most effective strategies for risk reduction.

This subchapter will explore practical smoking cessation strategies that can empower individuals to take control of their health and significantly lower their risk.

One effective approach to quitting smoking is to utilize a combination of behavioral therapies and pharmacological aids. Behavioral therapies, such as counseling sessions or support groups, help individuals understand their smoking triggers and develop coping strategies. Programs that focus on cognitive-behavioral techniques can assist in reshaping the thought patterns associated with smoking.

Pharmacological aids, including nicotine replacement therapies (NRTs) like patches, gums, or lozenges, can help manage withdrawal symptoms and reduce cravings. Combining these methods often leads to higher success rates, as they address both the physical and psychological components of nicotine addiction.

Setting a quit date can be a crucial step in the smoking cessation process. This date serves as a personal commitment and a target to work towards. It is advisable to choose a date within two weeks of making the decision to quit, allowing enough time to prepare without losing motivation. Individuals can mark this date on their calendars and plan the necessary steps leading up to it. Preparation may include removing cigarettes and smoking paraphernalia from their environment, informing friends and family for support, and identifying situations that may trigger the urge to smoke.

Another essential strategy for successfully quitting smoking is to develop a robust support network. Social support can significantly influence an individual's ability to quit. Friends, family members, or co-workers can provide encouragement and accountability. Additionally, joining a local or online support group can connect individuals with others facing similar challenges, creating a sense of community and shared experience. Many organizations also offer quitlines and resources that provide immediate assistance and motivation during difficult moments.

Finally, adopting healthy lifestyle changes can enhance the likelihood of successfully quitting smoking. Engaging in regular physical activity can reduce cravings and improve mood, while a balanced diet can help mitigate weight gain often associated with cessation.

Mindfulness practices, such as meditation and yoga, can also help manage stress and reduce the likelihood of relapse. By focusing on overall well-being, individuals can create a positive environment that supports their commitment to quitting smoking and ultimately reduces their risk of esophageal cancer. Through these strategies, individuals can take significant steps toward a healthier future, free from the dangers of tobacco.

# How To Reduce Esophageal Cancer Risk

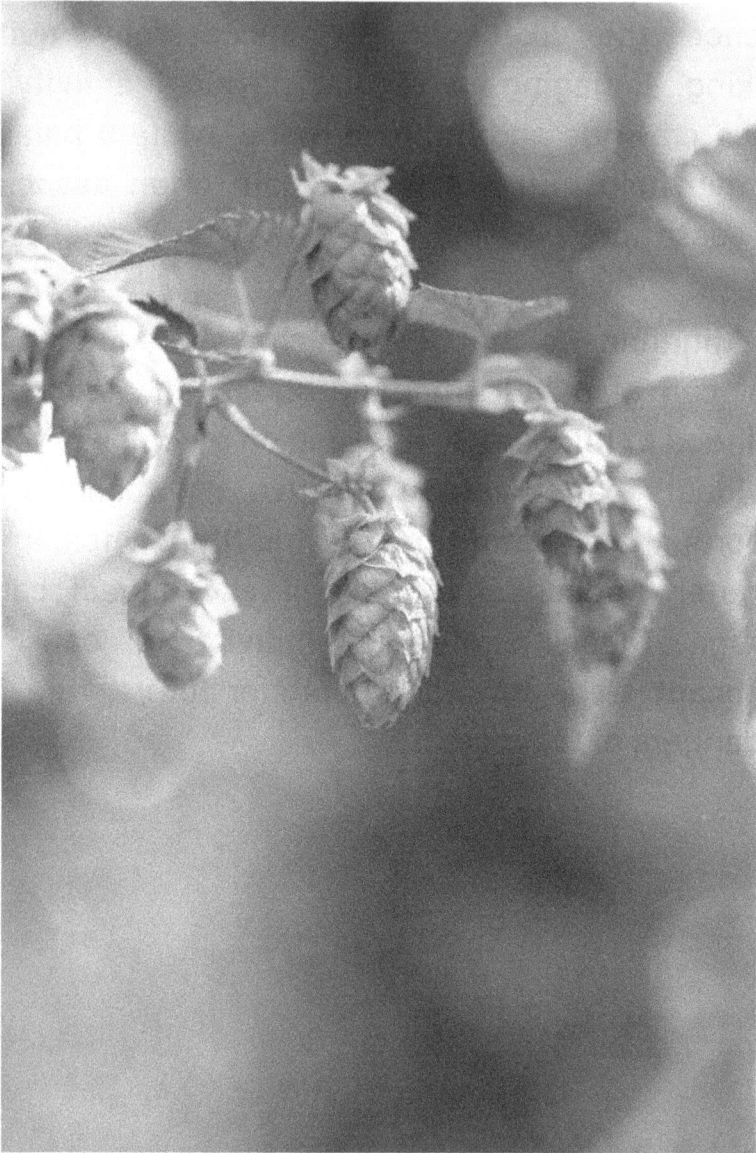

# Chapter 4

# Alcohol Consumption and Its Effects

## Understanding Alcohol as a Risk Factor

Alcohol consumption is a significant risk factor for esophageal cancer, a malignant condition that affects the esophagus, the tube connecting the throat to the stomach. Numerous studies have established a correlation between alcohol intake and an increased likelihood of developing this type of cancer, particularly squamous cell carcinoma and adenocarcinoma, the two main histological types.

The risk associated with alcohol is multifaceted, involving both the quantity and frequency of consumption, as well as individual susceptibility due to genetic and environmental factors.

The mechanism by which alcohol contributes to esophageal cancer is complex. Ethanol, the active component in alcoholic beverages, is metabolized in the liver and converted into acetaldehyde, a toxic compound that has been classified as a probable human carcinogen. Acetaldehyde can damage DNA and proteins, leading to mutations that may initiate the cancer development process.

Additionally, alcohol consumption can impair the body's ability to absorb essential nutrients, weaken the immune system, and exacerbate inflammation, all of which may further elevate cancer risk.

Research highlights a dose-response relationship between alcohol intake and esophageal cancer risk, meaning that the more alcohol a person consumes, the higher their risk. Moderate drinking may be associated with a lower risk compared to heavy drinking, but even moderate consumption is not without concern.

For individuals who have other risk factors, such as smoking or gastroesophageal reflux disease (GERD), even small amounts of alcohol can significantly increase the likelihood of developing esophageal cancer. This synergistic effect underscores the importance of assessing overall lifestyle choices when evaluating risk.

It is crucial for individuals concerned about esophageal cancer to understand their own drinking patterns and consider reducing or eliminating alcohol from their diets. Practical strategies to mitigate risk include setting clear limits on alcohol consumption, choosing alcohol-free days, and seeking support for lifestyle changes if needed.

For those who find it difficult to cut back, consulting healthcare professionals or joining support groups can provide valuable assistance in addressing alcohol use and exploring healthier alternatives.

In summary, understanding alcohol as a risk factor for esophageal cancer is vital for those focused on prevention. By recognizing the connection between alcohol consumption and cancer risk, individuals can make informed choices about their drinking habits. Reducing or eliminating alcohol intake not only contributes to lower cancer risk but also promotes overall health and well-being. As part of a comprehensive approach to risk reduction, addressing alcohol consumption should be a priority in the journey toward preventing esophageal cancer.

## Safe Drinking Guidelines

When it comes to reducing the risk of esophageal cancer, one critical aspect to consider is the consumption of beverages. The temperature, type, and frequency of what you drink can all play significant roles in influencing your esophageal health. Adhering to safe drinking guidelines can help mitigate risks associated with esophageal irritation and inflammation, which are potential precursors to cancer development. This subchapter outlines essential practices for choosing and consuming drinks in a way that supports esophageal well-being.

Firstly, temperature plays a vital role in the safety of your beverages. Research has indicated that drinking very hot liquids, particularly those exceeding 65 degrees Celsius (149 degrees Fahrenheit), may increase the risk of esophageal cancer. The high temperatures can cause thermal injury to the esophagus, leading to chronic inflammation and cellular changes.

To minimize this risk, allow hot drinks, such as tea or coffee, to cool down to a safe temperature before consumption. Aim for a drinking temperature that is comfortable and does not cause discomfort, generally around 55 degrees Celsius (131 degrees Fahrenheit) or lower.

In addition to temperature, the types of beverages you choose can impact your esophageal health. Alcohol consumption has been strongly linked to an increased risk of esophageal cancer, particularly in individuals who engage in heavy drinking or have a history of alcohol abuse. It is advisable to limit or avoid alcohol altogether.

If you choose to drink, moderation is key; the American Cancer Society recommends no more than one drink per day for women and two drinks per day for men. Opting for non-alcoholic alternatives such as herbal teas, water, or fresh fruit juices can be beneficial not only for reducing cancer risk but also for promoting overall health.

The consumption of sugary and acidic drinks should also be approached with caution. Beverages such as sodas, certain fruit juices, and energy drinks can contribute to gastroesophageal reflux disease (GERD), a condition that can exacerbate esophageal irritation and inflammation.

Individuals concerned about esophageal cancer should focus on hydration through plain water, which is not only safe but also essential for maintaining overall digestive health. If you enjoy flavored drinks, consider infusing water with fruits or herbs to create a healthy, refreshing alternative without the harmful effects of added sugars and acids.

Lastly, being mindful of drinking habits is crucial. Eating and drinking simultaneously can increase the likelihood of reflux symptoms, especially if large quantities are consumed. To support esophageal health, consider separating drinking from meals or limiting fluid intake during meals.

This practice can help reduce the pressure on the lower esophageal sphincter, minimizing the risk of acid reflux and its associated complications. Additionally, remaining upright for at least 30 minutes after eating can aid digestion and further protect the esophagus from potential irritants.

By following these safe drinking guidelines, individuals can take proactive steps toward reducing their risk of esophageal cancer. Combining mindful beverage choices with temperature considerations and drinking habits creates a comprehensive approach to esophageal health. Implementing these strategies not only fosters a healthier lifestyle but also empowers individuals to make informed decisions that contribute to long-term well-being.

## Alternatives to Alcohol

Alternatives to alcohol can play a significant role in reducing the risk of esophageal cancer, particularly for individuals seeking healthier lifestyle choices. Alcohol consumption has been linked to various types of cancer, including esophageal cancer, due to its ability to irritate the lining of the esophagus and its role in the formation of carcinogenic compounds. For those aiming to minimize their risk, exploring non-alcoholic beverages can be a beneficial strategy.

One popular alternative to traditional alcoholic drinks is non-alcoholic beer. Many breweries now offer a range of non-alcoholic options that maintain the flavors and social aspects of traditional beer without the harmful effects of alcohol.

These beverages typically contain minimal calories and may even provide some health benefits, such as antioxidants. Choosing non-alcoholic beer allows individuals to enjoy a familiar taste and experience while significantly reducing their cancer risk.

Another effective alternative is the use of sparkling water or flavored seltzers. These beverages offer a refreshing and hydrating option without the adverse effects associated with alcohol. Many brands infuse sparkling water with natural flavors, making them an appealing choice for those looking to enjoy a fizzy drink.

Additionally, seltzers can be mixed with fresh fruits or herbs to create unique mocktails, allowing individuals to engage in social drinking scenarios without alcohol.

Herbal teas represent another excellent alternative, providing a wide range of flavors and potential health benefits. Many herbal teas possess anti-inflammatory properties and contain antioxidants that may help protect against cancer.

Varieties such as green tea and chamomile not only offer soothing qualities but also promote overall well-being. By incorporating herbal teas into daily routines, individuals can replace alcoholic beverages with a nutritious option that supports esophageal health.

Lastly, juice and smoothie blends can serve as delicious alternatives to alcohol. Freshly squeezed juices or smoothies made from fruits and vegetables are packed with vitamins, minerals, and antioxidants. They promote a healthy lifestyle and can be tailored to individual preferences. By choosing these nutrient-rich options, individuals can satisfy their cravings for sweet or tangy flavors while steering clear of the risks associated with alcohol consumption.

In conclusion, exploring alternatives to alcohol is a proactive step individuals can take to reduce their risk of esophageal cancer. By opting for non-alcoholic beers, sparkling waters, herbal teas, and nutritious juices or smoothies, individuals can enjoy satisfying beverages without the health risks posed by alcohol. These choices not only contribute to a healthier lifestyle but also promote overall well-being, making them an essential part of a comprehensive approach to esophageal cancer prevention.

# How To Reduce Esophageal Cancer Risk

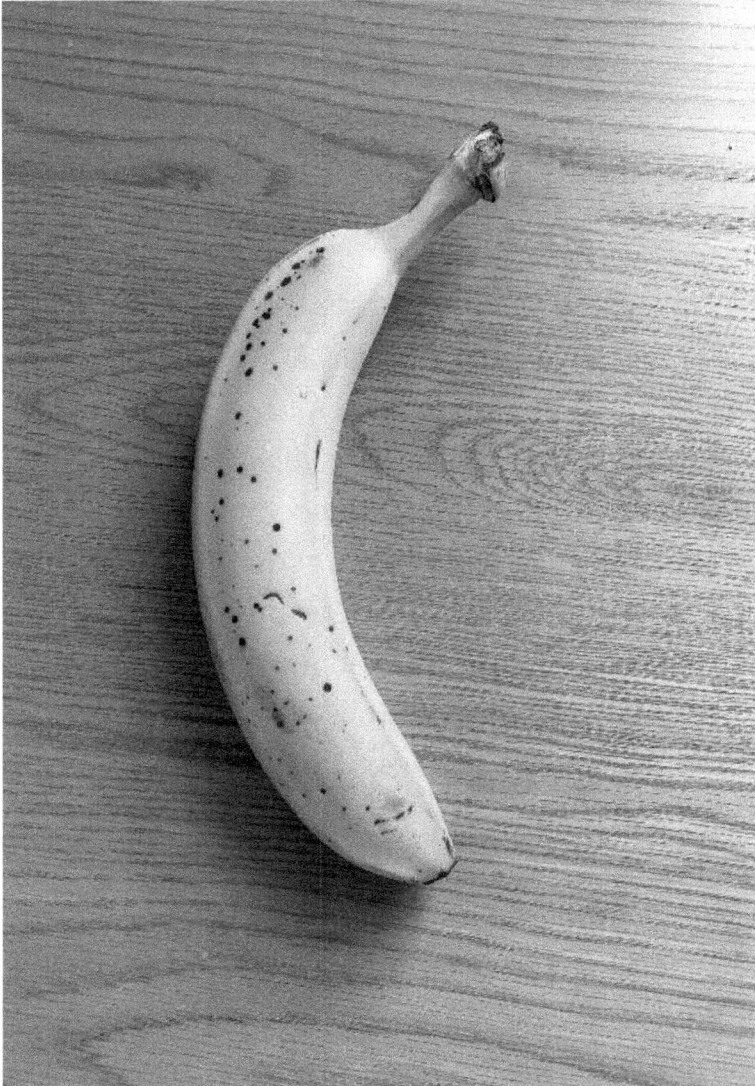

# Chapter 5

# Gastroesophageal Reflux Disease (GERD)

## Understanding GERD and Its Connection to Esophageal Cancer

Gastroesophageal reflux disease (GERD) is a chronic condition characterized by the backflow of stomach contents into the esophagus, leading to various symptoms such as heartburn, regurgitation, and difficulty swallowing. This condition occurs when the lower esophageal sphincter, a ring of muscle at the junction of the esophagus and stomach, fails to function properly.

Over time, persistent GERD can lead to inflammation and changes in the cells lining the esophagus, a condition known as esophagitis. Understanding GERD is crucial for individuals concerned about esophageal cancer, as the relationship between the two can significantly influence risk.

The connection between GERD and esophageal cancer, particularly esophageal adenocarcinoma, has been established through numerous studies. Chronic GERD can lead to Barrett's esophagus, a precancerous condition where the normal squamous cells of the esophagus are replaced by columnar cells. This cellular change increases the risk of developing esophageal cancer.

While Barrett's esophagus affects only a small percentage of those with GERD, the presence of this condition is a significant risk factor for esophageal adenocarcinoma. Therefore, individuals with frequent GERD symptoms should be vigilant and consider regular screenings, particularly if they experience chronic heartburn or have other risk factors.

Risk reduction strategies for individuals suffering from GERD are essential in minimizing the likelihood of progressing to more severe complications, including cancer. Lifestyle modifications, such as maintaining a healthy weight, avoiding trigger foods (like spicy or fatty meals), and not lying down immediately after eating, can help manage GERD symptoms.

Additionally, elevating the head during sleep and avoiding tight-fitting clothing can reduce pressure on the stomach, further alleviating reflux symptoms. These simple yet effective strategies can significantly improve quality of life and potentially lower the risk of esophageal cancer.

In some cases, medical intervention may be necessary for managing GERD effectively. Over-the-counter antacids, H2 receptor antagonists, and proton pump inhibitors (PPIs) are common medications that can help reduce stomach acid production, thereby relieving symptoms and preventing damage to the esophagus.

However, long-term use of PPIs has been associated with potential risks, including an increased likelihood of developing certain infections and nutrient deficiencies. It is vital for individuals to work closely with healthcare providers to determine the most appropriate treatment plan, balancing symptom relief with long-term health considerations.

Education and awareness are critical components in the fight against esophageal cancer. Individuals should be proactive in understanding their risk factors related to GERD and Barrett's esophagus. Regular medical check-ups, coupled with open discussions about symptoms and concerns, can lead to early detection and intervention if necessary.

By implementing effective lifestyle changes, seeking appropriate medical treatments, and staying informed, individuals can take significant steps toward reducing their risk of esophageal cancer while managing GERD effectively.

## Managing GERD Through Diet and Lifestyle

Managing gastroesophageal reflux disease (GERD) through diet and lifestyle changes is a crucial strategy for individuals concerned about the risk of esophageal cancer. GERD is characterized by the frequent backflow of stomach acid into the esophagus, which can lead to persistent inflammation and damage.

Over time, chronic GERD may increase the risk of Barrett's esophagus, a condition that can precede esophageal cancer. Therefore, understanding how to effectively manage GERD is essential for reducing cancer risk.

Diet plays a pivotal role in managing GERD symptoms. Individuals should focus on incorporating a variety of low-acid foods into their meals. Foods such as oatmeal, bananas, melons, and green leafy vegetables can help neutralize stomach acid.

Additionally, lean proteins such as chicken and fish, as well as whole grains, are less likely to trigger reflux compared to fatty or fried foods. It is also important to limit the intake of known trigger foods, which can vary from person to person but often include spicy dishes, citrus fruits, chocolate, and caffeinated beverages.

In addition to dietary choices, meal timing and portion size significantly influence GERD management. Individuals are advised to eat smaller, more frequent meals rather than large portions, which can increase abdominal pressure and exacerbate reflux. Moreover, avoiding late-night meals is beneficial; allowing at least two to three hours between the last meal and bedtime can reduce the likelihood of nighttime reflux episodes.

Adapting eating habits to include mindful eating practices—such as chewing thoroughly and eating slowly—can also contribute to better digestion and reduced symptoms.

Lifestyle modifications beyond diet are equally important in managing GERD. Maintaining a healthy weight is crucial, as excess body weight can increase abdominal pressure and exacerbate reflux symptoms. For individuals who are overweight, even modest weight loss can significantly alleviate GERD symptoms.

Additionally, elevating the head of the bed by six to eight inches can help prevent nighttime symptoms by using gravity to keep stomach acid from flowing back into the esophagus during sleep. Regular physical activity also supports weight management and overall digestive health, but individuals should avoid vigorous exercise immediately after meals.

Finally, it is essential to recognize the impact of certain habits and substances on GERD management. Smoking and excessive alcohol consumption can worsen reflux symptoms and should be avoided. For those who find it challenging to quit smoking or reduce alcohol intake, seeking professional help or support groups may be beneficial.

Stress management techniques, such as yoga, meditation, and deep-breathing exercises, can also aid in reducing GERD symptoms, as stress can exacerbate acid reflux. By implementing these dietary and lifestyle strategies, individuals can take proactive steps toward managing GERD effectively, ultimately reducing their risk of esophageal cancer.

## When to Seek Medical Advice

When it comes to esophageal cancer, early detection and intervention can significantly influence outcomes. For individuals concerned about their health and the potential risk of developing this type of cancer, understanding when to seek medical advice is crucial. This subchapter aims to equip readers with the knowledge necessary to recognize potential warning signs and symptoms, as well as the importance of regular screenings, particularly for those at higher risk.

One of the primary indicators that may warrant medical consultation is the presence of persistent symptoms that are often associated with esophageal issues. Individuals should pay attention to symptoms such as difficulty swallowing (dysphagia), unexplained weight loss, or persistent heartburn that does not respond to over-the-counter medications. These signs may not necessarily indicate cancer, but they can signify underlying conditions that require further investigation. If these symptoms persist for more than a few weeks, it is essential to schedule an appointment with a healthcare professional for a thorough evaluation.

For those who fall into higher-risk categories, such as individuals with a history of gastroesophageal reflux disease (GERD), Barrett's esophagus, or a family history of esophageal cancer, the need for proactive medical advice becomes even more critical. Regular surveillance, including endoscopic procedures, may be recommended to monitor any cellular changes in the esophagus. Understanding personal risk factors can empower individuals to engage in conversations with their healthcare providers about appropriate screening schedules and preventive measures tailored to their specific circumstances.

In addition to recognizing symptoms, individuals should be aware of lifestyle factors that may increase their risk of esophageal cancer. Heavy alcohol consumption, tobacco use, obesity, and diets high in processed meats and low in fruits and vegetables can all contribute to increased risk. If individuals find themselves engaged in these behaviors, it may be beneficial to seek guidance on lifestyle modifications and risk reduction strategies. Healthcare professionals can offer personalized advice on nutrition, weight management, and smoking cessation, all of which are vital components in mitigating esophageal cancer risk.

Finally, it is important to cultivate a proactive approach to health. Routine check-ups and open communication with healthcare providers can foster a partnership geared towards prevention. Individuals should feel empowered to voice their concerns and ask questions regarding their risk of esophageal cancer. By remaining vigilant and informed, individuals can take significant steps toward reducing their risk and advocating for their health, ultimately enhancing their quality of life and well-being.

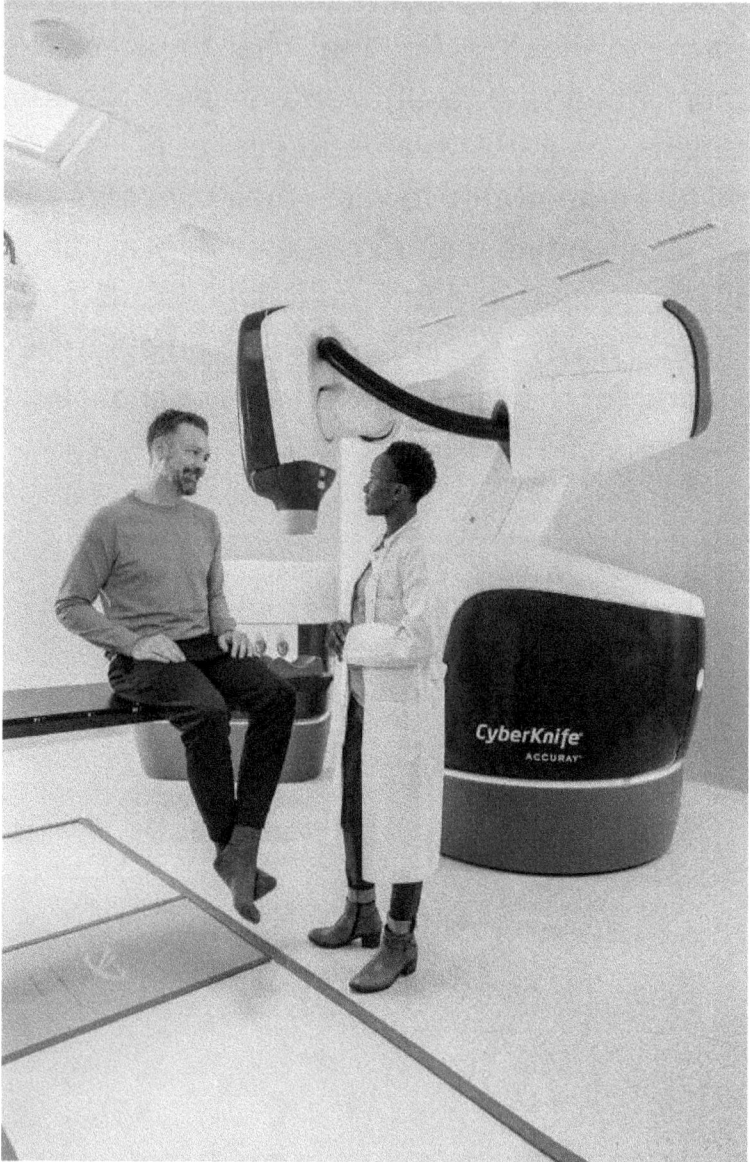

# Chapter 6

# Regular Screenings and Medical Care

## The Importance of Regular Check-ups

Regular check-ups play a crucial role in the early detection and prevention of esophageal cancer, making them an essential component of any risk reduction strategy. For individuals concerned about their health and specifically about esophageal cancer, understanding the significance of these medical evaluations is vital.

During these appointments, healthcare providers can assess risk factors, monitor symptoms, and recommend preventive measures tailored to individual needs. This proactive approach not only helps in catching potential issues early but also empowers individuals to take charge of their health.

One of the primary advantages of regular check-ups is the opportunity for personalized risk assessment. Factors such as age, family history, lifestyle choices, and pre-existing conditions contribute to an individual's overall risk for esophageal cancer.

Healthcare professionals can analyze these elements during check-ups and provide informed advice on how to mitigate risks. This may include lifestyle modifications, dietary changes, or even screening recommendations for those at higher risk. By having these conversations, individuals can gain a clearer understanding of their health status and the steps they can take to reduce their risk.

Furthermore, regular check-ups facilitate the early detection of potential precursors to esophageal cancer, such as Barrett's esophagus, a condition that arises from chronic acid reflux. This condition can increase the risk of developing esophageal cancer if left unmonitored.

Through procedures like endoscopies, doctors can identify changes in the esophagus that may signal the onset of Barrett's esophagus and implement appropriate management strategies. Early intervention not only enhances treatment outcomes but also significantly improves survival rates, underscoring the importance of staying vigilant about one's health.

Additionally, routine check-ups provide an opportunity for healthcare providers to educate patients about the latest research and advancements in esophageal cancer prevention. This information can be invaluable, as new findings may lead to updated guidelines on diet, exercise, and other lifestyle factors that influence cancer risk.

By staying informed through regular visits, individuals can adapt their health strategies in accordance with the latest evidence, ensuring they are utilizing the most effective methods for reducing their risk of esophageal cancer.

In conclusion, the importance of regular check-ups cannot be overstated for those concerned about esophageal cancer. These appointments serve as a vital mechanism for personalized risk assessment, early detection of potential health issues, and ongoing education about prevention strategies.

By prioritizing these check-ups, individuals can significantly increase their chances of catching problems early and making informed decisions about their health, thereby reducing their overall risk of esophageal cancer. Taking proactive steps today can lead to a healthier tomorrow, making regular medical evaluations an indispensable part of any cancer prevention plan.

## Screening Options for High-Risk Individuals

Screening options for high-risk individuals are critical for early detection and prevention of esophageal cancer. Certain factors, including age, lifestyle choices, and underlying medical conditions, can significantly increase an individual's risk.

For those who fall into high-risk categories, proactive screening measures can lead to early intervention, which is essential for improving outcomes. Understanding the available screening methods and their importance is a vital step in managing personal health and reducing the risk of esophageal cancer.

One common screening method for high-risk individuals is endoscopy, which allows doctors to visualize the esophagus directly. During this procedure, a thin, flexible tube with a camera is inserted through the throat, enabling the examination of the esophageal lining.

Endoscopy is particularly valuable for individuals with Barrett's esophagus, a condition that arises from chronic gastroesophageal reflux disease (GERD) and is associated with an increased risk of esophageal cancer. Regular endoscopic surveillance can help detect precancerous changes early, facilitating timely treatment and potentially preventing the progression to cancer.

Another important screening tool is the use of biopsies during endoscopy. If any abnormal tissue is observed, a biopsy can be performed to analyze the cells for signs of dysplasia or malignancy. This histological evaluation is crucial, as it provides definitive information about the presence and extent of cancerous changes.

For those with a family history of esophageal cancer or other risk factors, regular biopsies can be a proactive measure to monitor for early signs of the disease, allowing for intervention before cancer develops.

In addition to endoscopy, imaging techniques such as endoscopic ultrasound (EUS) can be employed to assess the depth of tumor invasion and the involvement of nearby lymph nodes. EUS is particularly beneficial for guiding treatment decisions, as it provides detailed information about the staging of esophageal cancer. For those at high risk, discussing the potential benefits of EUS with a healthcare provider can lead to more informed choices regarding screening and surveillance strategies.

Overall, maintaining an open dialogue with healthcare professionals about personal risk factors is essential for determining the most appropriate screening options. Individuals concerned about esophageal cancer should engage in regular check-ups and discuss their specific risk profiles.

By taking an active role in their health care, high-risk individuals can benefit from tailored screening strategies that not only aim to detect early-stage cancer but also empower them with knowledge and resources to effectively reduce their risk of esophageal cancer.

## Communicating with Your Healthcare Provider

Effective communication with your healthcare provider is a critical component in the journey toward reducing the risk of esophageal cancer. Many individuals who are concerned about their health may feel overwhelmed by the myriad of information available, leading to uncertainty about how to approach discussions with their medical team.

Building a relationship characterized by open dialogue and trust can empower patients to take proactive steps in managing their health. By fostering clear communication, individuals can better understand their risks and the preventive measures they can undertake.

To initiate meaningful conversations, it is essential to come prepared for your medical appointments. Before your visit, compile a list of questions and concerns related to esophageal cancer risk factors, symptoms, and preventive strategies. Consider your personal health history, including any symptoms such as difficulty swallowing, heartburn, or weight loss, as these details can provide your healthcare provider with valuable context.

Additionally, keep a record of any medications or supplements you are taking, as these can influence your overall risk profile. By organizing your thoughts and concerns ahead of time, you can ensure that your dialogue with your provider is focused and productive.

During your appointment, actively engage in the conversation. Don't hesitate to voice your concerns or seek clarification on terms that may be unfamiliar. It is important to understand the significance of factors such as gastroesophageal reflux disease (GERD), Barrett's esophagus, and lifestyle choices like smoking and diet, which can contribute to esophageal cancer risk.

If your provider recommends specific screenings or tests, ask about the rationale behind these suggestions and how they fit into a broader prevention strategy. A collaborative approach will help you feel more informed and confident in your healthcare decisions.

Follow-up after your appointment is equally crucial in maintaining effective communication. If you receive test results or recommendations, ensure that you understand the next steps. If anything is unclear, don't hesitate to reach out to your healthcare provider for further explanation.

Additionally, consider scheduling regular check-ups to monitor your health and discuss any new developments or concerns that may arise. This ongoing dialogue not only reinforces the importance of preventative care but also demonstrates your commitment to managing your health proactively.

Finally, consider broadening your support network by involving family members or friends in your healthcare discussions. They can provide emotional support and help you remember important information or questions to ask during your appointments. Moreover, having someone accompany you can facilitate a more comprehensive understanding of the conversation with your provider. Encouraging open communication about esophageal cancer not only aids your personal risk reduction strategies but can also foster awareness and support within your community, ultimately contributing to a broader culture of health and prevention.

# How To Reduce Esophageal Cancer Risk

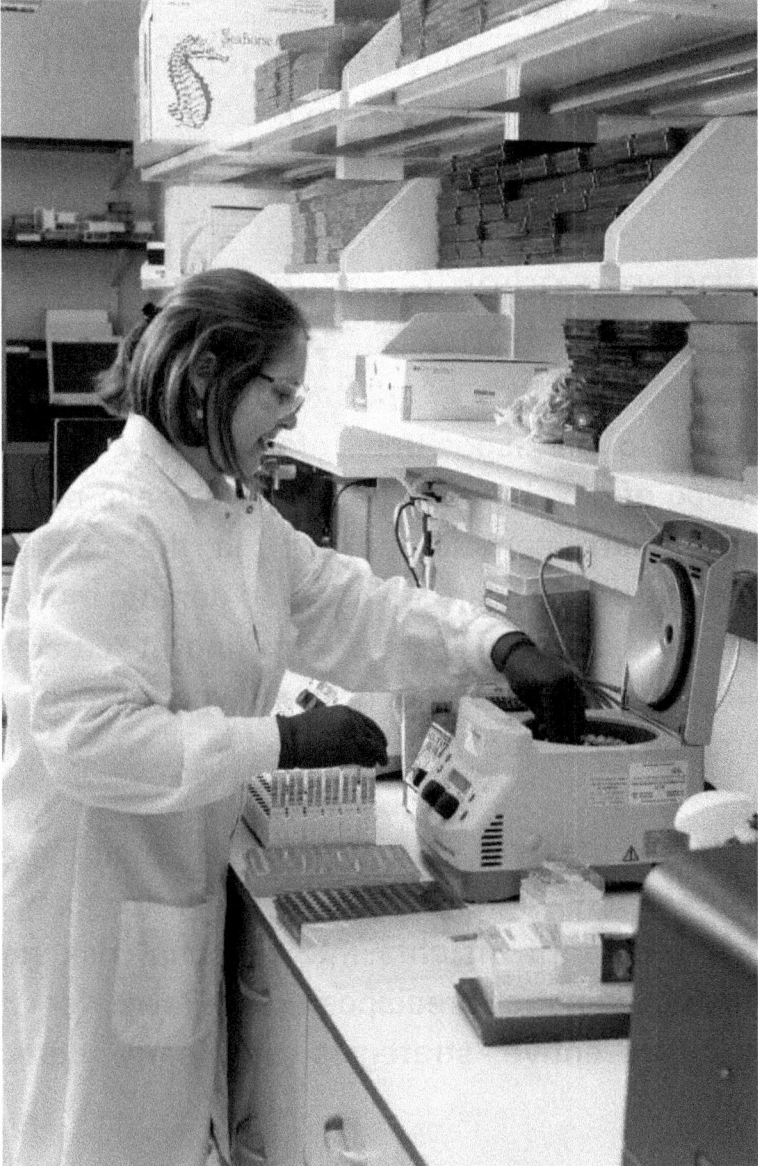

# Chapter 7

# Genetic Factors and Family History

## Understanding Genetic Predisposition

Genetic predisposition refers to the increased likelihood of developing a particular disease based on an individual's genetic makeup. In the context of esophageal cancer, certain inherited genetic mutations can elevate a person's risk, making it crucial for individuals concerned about this type of cancer to understand these factors.

While lifestyle choices and environmental exposures play significant roles, genetics can also provide important insights into personal risk levels. Identifying genetic predisposition allows for more tailored preventive strategies and early detection measures.

Several genes have been implicated in esophageal cancer, including TP53, CDKN2A, and others that may influence cellular growth and repair mechanisms. Mutations in these genes can disrupt normal cellular function, leading to uncontrolled cell proliferation, which is a hallmark of cancer.

Although the majority of esophageal cancer cases arise sporadically, understanding the genetic factors involved can help individuals assess their risk and make informed decisions about surveillance and prevention strategies. Genetic testing can be a valuable tool for those with a family history of esophageal cancer or related conditions, allowing for early intervention when necessary.

In addition to specific gene mutations, certain inherited conditions, such as Barrett's esophagus, can significantly increase the risk of developing esophageal cancer. Barrett's esophagus occurs when the cells lining the esophagus undergo changes due to prolonged exposure to stomach acid, often as a result of gastroesophageal reflux disease (GERD).

Individuals with Barrett's esophagus have a greater likelihood of developing esophageal adenocarcinoma, a common subtype of esophageal cancer. Understanding these conditions and their genetic links is vital for individuals who may be at risk, as it can prompt proactive health screenings and lifestyle modifications.

It's important to note that having a genetic predisposition does not guarantee the development of esophageal cancer; rather, it indicates an increased risk. Environmental factors, such as diet, smoking, and alcohol consumption, can also interact with genetic predispositions to influence cancer risk.

Individuals who are aware of their genetic background can take proactive measures to mitigate these risks through lifestyle changes, regular medical check-ups, and informed discussions with healthcare providers about personalized screening protocols.

In conclusion, understanding genetic predisposition is a key component of comprehensive esophageal cancer risk reduction. By recognizing the interplay between genetics and environmental factors, individuals can better equip themselves with knowledge and strategies to lower their risk.

Engaging in genetic counseling, considering genetic testing when appropriate, and maintaining an open dialogue with healthcare professionals about personal risk factors can empower individuals to take control of their health and make informed decisions that may ultimately reduce their risk of esophageal cancer.

## When to Consider Genetic Testing

When to consider genetic testing is a critical decision for individuals concerned about esophageal cancer and seeking practical strategies for risk reduction. Genetic testing can provide valuable insights into one's predisposition to certain cancers, including esophageal cancer.

It is important to understand the circumstances under which testing is beneficial, as well as the implications of the results. Individuals with a family history of esophageal cancer or related gastrointestinal cancers should be particularly vigilant, as hereditary factors can significantly increase risk.

Individuals experiencing symptoms such as difficulty swallowing, persistent heartburn, or unexplained weight loss should also contemplate genetic testing. These symptoms may indicate underlying conditions that could be linked to an increased risk of esophageal cancer.

Discussing these concerns with a healthcare provider can help determine if genetic testing is appropriate. In cases where family members have been diagnosed with esophageal cancer or related conditions, testing can reveal specific genetic mutations that may inform personalized prevention strategies.

Another key factor to consider is the presence of known genetic syndromes in the family. Conditions such as Lynch syndrome, which increases the risk of several cancers, including esophageal cancer, warrant serious consideration for genetic testing. For those with a personal or family history of such syndromes, understanding one's genetic makeup can guide decisions about surveillance, preventive measures, and lifestyle modifications that may help reduce cancer risk.

Furthermore, individuals of certain ethnic backgrounds, such as those of Ashkenazi Jewish descent, may have a higher likelihood of carrying specific genetic mutations associated with cancer. For these individuals, proactive genetic testing can be an essential step in assessing cancer risk.

Engaging with genetic counselors can provide clarity on testing options, potential outcomes, and the emotional impact of results, enabling individuals to make informed decisions about their health.

Ultimately, genetic testing should be seen as one component of a comprehensive risk reduction strategy for esophageal cancer. By integrating genetic insights with lifestyle changes, dietary adjustments, and regular screenings, individuals can take a proactive stance toward their health. Understanding when to pursue genetic testing empowers individuals to make informed choices about their cancer risk, fostering a sense of control in the face of uncertainty.

## Family History and Risk Assessment

Family history plays a pivotal role in the risk assessment of esophageal cancer, as certain hereditary factors can significantly influence an individual's likelihood of developing this disease. Understanding one's family medical history is essential for identifying potential risks. Individuals with a family background of esophageal cancer or related conditions, such as Barrett's esophagus or gastroesophageal reflux disease (GERD), should be particularly vigilant.

Family history can often serve as a warning sign, prompting early screening and proactive lifestyle changes. By gathering detailed information about relatives' health issues, individuals can gain valuable insights into their own risk factors.

Genetic predispositions are part of the broader picture when it comes to family history and esophageal cancer risk. Certain inherited syndromes, such as Lynch syndrome or familial adenomatous polyposis, may increase susceptibility to various types of cancer, including esophageal cancer.

Individuals who suspect they may have such genetic conditions should consider genetic counseling and testing. Understanding whether these genetic markers are present can guide preventive measures and inform healthcare providers about the best strategies for monitoring and managing risk.

# How To Reduce Esophageal Cancer Risk

Lifestyle factors, often intertwined with family history, further complicate risk assessment. For instance, habits such as smoking, excessive alcohol consumption, and poor dietary choices can exacerbate the likelihood of developing esophageal cancer, especially in those with a familial tendency. It is crucial for individuals to evaluate their lifestyle in the context of their family history.

For example, if multiple family members have struggled with obesity or gastroesophageal reflux disease, it may indicate a hereditary propensity that can be addressed through lifestyle modifications. Emphasizing a balanced diet, regular exercise, and quitting smoking can help mitigate these risks.

Regular screenings and medical check-ups are vital for those with a concerning family history of esophageal cancer. Early detection can make a significant difference in treatment outcomes. Individuals should discuss their family history with healthcare providers to determine appropriate screening schedules and tests.

This proactive approach not only aids in catching potential issues early but also empowers individuals to take charge of their health. Educating oneself about the signs and symptoms of esophageal cancer can also enhance awareness, leading to timely medical consultations when necessary.

In summary, understanding family history is crucial in assessing the risk of esophageal cancer. By recognizing the interplay between genetic predispositions, lifestyle choices, and familial patterns, individuals can take informed steps toward risk reduction. Engaging in open conversations with family members about health histories, consulting healthcare professionals for personalized risk assessments, and adopting healthier lifestyle practices are all essential strategies. Through these measures, individuals can significantly lower their risk and enhance their overall well-being, paving the way for a healthier future.

# How To Reduce Esophageal Cancer Risk

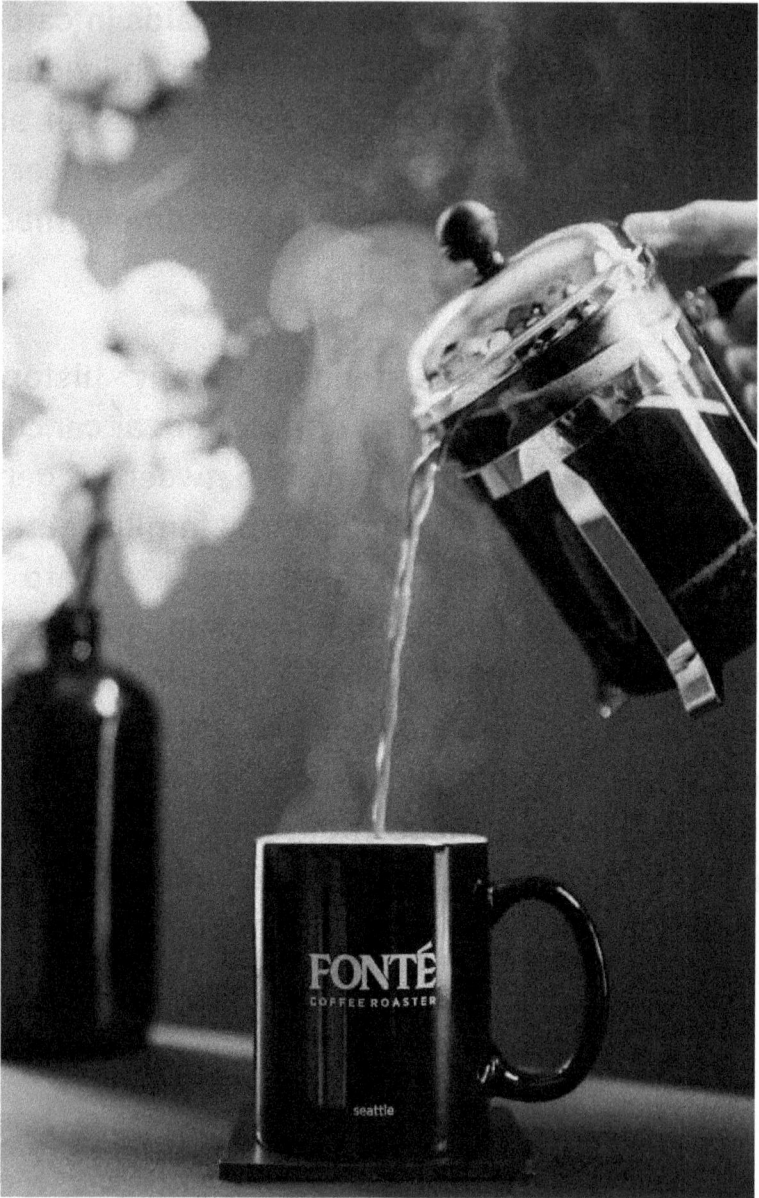

A Comprehensive Guide

# Chapter 8

# Environmental and Occupational Risks

## Identifying Environmental Risk Factors

Identifying environmental risk factors is a crucial step in understanding and reducing the risk of esophageal cancer. Environmental factors encompass a wide range of influences, from exposure to certain chemicals and pollutants to lifestyle choices that can affect overall health.

By recognizing these risks, individuals can take proactive measures to mitigate their exposure and improve their chances of preventing this disease. This subchapter aims to illuminate the key environmental factors linked to esophageal cancer and provide actionable strategies to reduce risk.

One significant environmental risk factor is the consumption of certain foods and beverages. High-temperature foods and drinks, particularly when consumed frequently, have been associated with an increased risk of esophageal cancer. The practice of drinking very hot beverages, such as tea or coffee, can lead to thermal injury to the esophagus, which may promote cellular changes over time.

Additionally, a diet high in processed foods, red meats, and low in fruits and vegetables can contribute to overall health deterioration and, consequently, increase cancer risk. To minimize these risks, individuals should consider adopting a diet rich in whole foods, emphasizing fruits, vegetables, and whole grains while limiting the intake of processed and high-temperature items.

Another critical factor is the exposure to certain chemicals and pollutants in the environment. Occupational exposure to substances such as asbestos, certain industrial chemicals, and even secondhand smoke has been linked to a heightened risk of esophageal cancer.

Individuals who work in industries such as construction, manufacturing, or agriculture should be particularly vigilant about their exposure to these harmful substances. Proper protective measures, such as wearing appropriate safety gear and following workplace safety protocols, can significantly reduce these risks.

Furthermore, reducing exposure to environmental tobacco smoke in public and private spaces is essential for non-smokers, especially those living with smokers.

Socioeconomic status also plays a role in environmental risk factors for esophageal cancer. Individuals from lower socioeconomic backgrounds may have limited access to healthcare, nutritious foods, and health education, which can contribute to higher cancer rates. Moreover, living in areas with high pollution levels can exacerbate health disparities. Community engagement and advocacy for cleaner environments, better healthcare access, and nutritional education are vital strategies for addressing these disparities.

Individuals can support local initiatives aimed at improving air quality and access to healthy foods, which can collectively contribute to cancer risk reduction.

Lastly, understanding the impact of lifestyle choices, such as alcohol consumption and smoking, is essential in identifying environmental risk factors. Heavy alcohol consumption has been strongly correlated with esophageal cancer, particularly in individuals who also smoke. The combination of these two risk factors significantly increases the likelihood of developing this disease.

To combat these risks, individuals should be encouraged to limit alcohol intake and seek support for smoking cessation. Health professionals can play a pivotal role in providing resources and support for those looking to make these lifestyle changes, ultimately contributing to a lower risk of esophageal cancer.

In conclusion, identifying environmental risk factors is a fundamental aspect of esophageal cancer prevention. By understanding the influence of dietary habits, chemical exposures, socioeconomic status, and lifestyle choices, individuals can implement practical strategies to reduce their risk. Awareness and proactive measures can empower individuals to take control of their health and contribute to a broader impact on community well-being. As we continue to explore the pathways to risk reduction, recognizing and addressing these environmental factors will be pivotal in the fight against esophageal cancer.

## Occupational Hazards and Esophageal Cancer

Occupational hazards play a significant role in the risk of developing various types of cancer, including esophageal cancer. Understanding the connection between certain occupations and the likelihood of this disease can inform individuals about potential risks and help them adopt preventive measures. This subchapter aims to shed light on the occupational factors associated with esophageal cancer and provide practical strategies for risk reduction.

Certain occupations are known to expose workers to carcinogenic substances that can contribute to the development of esophageal cancer. For example, individuals working in industries such as metalworking, construction, and textile manufacturing may come into contact with harmful chemicals, asbestos, and dust that can irritate the esophagus.

Additionally, workers in the food and beverage industry, particularly those involved in high-heat cooking methods or exposure to smoke, may face increased risks due to thermal injury and carcinogenic compounds present in charred foods. Recognizing these occupational hazards is the first step toward mitigating risk.

Implementing safety measures in the workplace is essential for reducing exposure to harmful substances. Workers should be encouraged to use personal protective equipment (PPE), such as masks and gloves, when handling chemicals or working in environments with potential carcinogens.

Employers can also play a crucial role by providing training on safe handling practices and ensuring that ventilation systems are in place to minimize airborne contaminants. Regular health screenings and monitoring for early signs of esophageal issues can further aid in early detection and intervention.

For individuals concerned about their occupational exposure, it is advisable to seek positions that prioritize health and safety standards. This may involve researching companies' safety records, advocating for better workplace conditions, or even considering career transitions into fields with lower associated cancer risks.

Those already in high-risk occupations should engage in proactive health management, including regular medical check-ups and discussions with healthcare professionals about potential risks related to their work environment.

In addition to workplace safety, adopting a lifestyle that supports esophageal health can further reduce risk. This includes maintaining a balanced diet rich in fruits and vegetables, avoiding excessive alcohol consumption, and quitting smoking if applicable. Individuals should also be mindful of their weight and engage in regular physical activity, as obesity has been linked to an increased risk of esophageal cancer.

By combining workplace safety measures with healthy lifestyle choices, individuals can create a comprehensive approach to reducing their risk of esophageal cancer.

## Mitigating Environmental Risks

Mitigating environmental risks is a crucial aspect of reducing the likelihood of esophageal cancer, particularly for individuals who are proactive about their health. The environment plays a significant role in our overall well-being, and certain environmental factors can increase the risk of developing this form of cancer.

By understanding these risks and implementing strategies to mitigate them, individuals can take meaningful steps toward protecting themselves.

One of the primary environmental factors linked to esophageal cancer is exposure to harmful chemicals and pollutants. Air quality, for instance, can significantly influence cancer risk. Individuals living in areas with high levels of pollution, such as industrial regions or cities with heavy traffic, may be at an increased risk.

To mitigate this risk, it is essential to stay informed about local air quality reports and take precautions during days when pollution levels are high. This could include limiting outdoor activities or using air purifiers indoors to reduce exposure to airborne toxins.

Another critical area of concern is the consumption of certain foods and beverages that may be contaminated with carcinogens. For example, processed meats and foods cooked at high temperatures, especially those charred or smoked, can produce harmful compounds.

Individuals can reduce their risk by making informed dietary choices, opting for whole, unprocessed foods, and employing healthier cooking methods such as steaming or baking instead of frying or grilling at high temperatures.

Additionally, being mindful of food sources and supporting local, organic farms can help minimize exposure to pesticides and other harmful chemicals.

Water quality also plays a significant role in environmental health. Contaminated drinking water can contain various carcinogens, including heavy metals and chemical pollutants. Individuals should consider testing their water supply, especially if they live in older homes with outdated plumbing.

Installing water filtration systems can further reduce exposure to harmful substances. Staying informed about local water quality reports and advocating for clean water initiatives can also contribute to a healthier community and reduced cancer risk.

Lastly, reducing exposure to tobacco smoke, both directly and indirectly, is essential in mitigating environmental risks associated with esophageal cancer. Secondhand smoke contains numerous carcinogens that can increase the risk of various cancers, including esophageal cancer. Individuals can take steps to create smoke-free environments in their homes and advocate for smoke-free policies in public spaces. Supporting cessation programs for smokers and promoting awareness about the dangers of tobacco use further contribute to reducing environmental risks not just for individuals, but for the community as a whole.

In summary, mitigating environmental risks associated with esophageal cancer requires a multifaceted approach. By being aware of air and water quality, making informed dietary choices, and advocating for smoke-free environments, individuals can significantly reduce their exposure to potential carcinogens. Taking proactive steps not only protects personal health but also fosters a healthier environment for all, ultimately contributing to the broader goal of cancer prevention.

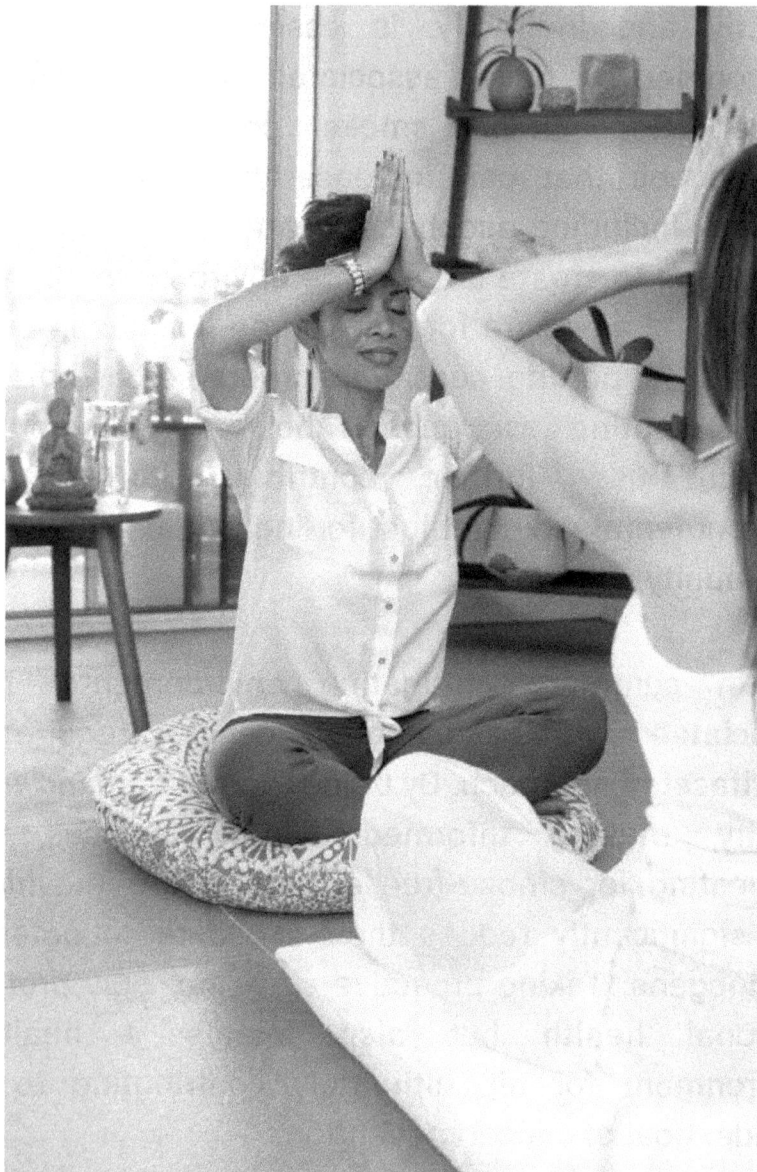

# Chapter 9

# Psychological Well-Being and Stress Management

## The Connection Between Stress and Cancer Risk

The relationship between stress and cancer risk is a topic of increasing interest in the field of health research, particularly in the context of esophageal cancer. Stress, both chronic and acute, can influence various physiological processes in the body, potentially leading to an elevated risk of developing cancer.

Understanding how stress affects cancer risk is crucial for individuals concerned about esophageal cancer, as it provides insights into additional lifestyle modifications that can contribute to risk reduction.

Chronic stress triggers a cascade of biological responses, including the release of stress hormones such as cortisol and adrenaline. These hormones, while essential for the body's fight-or-flight response, can have detrimental effects when elevated over prolonged periods.

Research suggests that chronic stress may lead to inflammation, a known factor in cancer development. Inflammation can damage DNA and promote the proliferation of cancerous cells, making it particularly pertinent to esophageal cancer, where chronic irritation and inflammation of the esophagus can lead to precancerous conditions such as Barrett's esophagus.

Moreover, stress can influence lifestyle choices that further increase cancer risk. Individuals under stress may resort to unhealthy coping mechanisms, such as smoking, excessive alcohol consumption, or poor dietary choices. These behaviors are not only detrimental to overall health but are also established risk factors for esophageal cancer.

For example, smoking is a significant contributor to esophageal squamous cell carcinoma, and heavy alcohol use has been linked to both squamous cell carcinoma and adenocarcinoma of the esophagus. Therefore, managing stress effectively can lead to healthier lifestyle choices, thereby potentially reducing cancer risk.

The psychological impact of stress also plays a role in health behaviors. Stress can lead to fatigue, decreased motivation, and a sense of helplessness, all of which can hinder individuals from engaging in preventive health measures.

Regular screenings, maintaining a healthy weight, and adhering to a balanced diet rich in fruits and vegetables are vital strategies for esophageal cancer prevention. By implementing stress management techniques, individuals can enhance their mental well-being, making it easier to pursue these proactive health behaviors.

Incorporating stress-reduction strategies into daily life can be a practical approach for those seeking to lower their risk of esophageal cancer. Techniques such as mindfulness meditation, physical activity, and social support systems can significantly mitigate the effects of stress.

Practicing relaxation methods not only improves mental health but also has positive implications for physical health, potentially decreasing the risk of cancer. By understanding the connection between stress and cancer risk, individuals can take actionable steps toward a healthier lifestyle that promotes both emotional resilience and physical well-being.

## Techniques for Stress Reduction

Stress plays a significant role in overall health, and its management is crucial for individuals concerned about esophageal cancer. Research indicates that chronic stress can negatively impact immune function and may contribute to the development of various cancers, including esophageal cancer.

Therefore, adopting effective stress reduction techniques can not only enhance well-being but also serve as a preventive measure against potential health issues. This subchapter explores practical strategies that individuals can implement to mitigate stress and reduce their risk of esophageal cancer.

Mindfulness and meditation are powerful techniques that can help individuals cope with stress. Mindfulness involves focusing on the present moment while acknowledging and accepting one's feelings and thoughts without judgment.

Regular practice of mindfulness meditation can lead to significant reductions in stress and anxiety levels. Individuals can start by dedicating just a few minutes each day to mindfulness exercises, such as deep breathing, body scans, or guided imagery. These practices can help cultivate a sense of calm and promote emotional resilience, which is vital for maintaining overall health.

Physical activity is another effective way to reduce stress and enhance overall well-being. Engaging in regular exercise releases endorphins, which are natural mood lifters. Activities like walking, jogging, yoga, or even dancing can not only reduce stress but also improve cardiovascular health and aid in weight management—factors that contribute to esophageal cancer risk.

Aim for at least 150 minutes of moderate-intensity aerobic activity each week, complemented by strength training exercises. Finding a form of exercise that is enjoyable can increase adherence to a routine and provide additional motivation to stay active in the long term.

Social support plays a critical role in stress management. Building and maintaining strong relationships with family, friends, or support groups can provide individuals with a network of encouragement during challenging times. Open communication about fears and concerns can alleviate stress and foster a sense of belonging.

Participating in community activities or support groups focused on health and wellness can also provide valuable resources and coping strategies. Engaging with others who share similar concerns can create a supportive environment that promotes proactive health management.

Lastly, cultivating healthy lifestyle habits, such as proper nutrition and sufficient sleep, can significantly impact stress levels. A balanced diet rich in fruits, vegetables, whole grains, and lean proteins can support physical health and improve mood. Additionally, prioritizing sleep hygiene—establishing a regular sleep schedule, creating a restful environment, and limiting screen time before bed—can enhance sleep quality and reduce stress.

Together, these lifestyle modifications can contribute to a robust defense against stress and its potential impact on esophageal cancer risk. By integrating these techniques into daily life, individuals can take proactive steps toward both stress reduction and cancer prevention.

## Building a Support System

Building a support system is an essential aspect of reducing the risk of esophageal cancer, as it fosters an environment of shared knowledge, emotional strength, and practical assistance. For individuals concerned about their health and well-being, having a network of support can enhance the effectiveness of risk reduction efforts.

This subchapter will explore the various ways to create a robust support system that empowers individuals to take proactive steps in preventing esophageal cancer.

First and foremost, connecting with healthcare professionals is crucial in building a support system. Regular consultations with doctors, dietitians, and oncologists can provide individuals with personalized advice and strategies tailored to their specific health needs. Healthcare professionals can offer insights into risk factors associated with esophageal cancer and recommend lifestyle changes that can mitigate these risks.

Establishing open lines of communication with these experts ensures that individuals stay informed about the latest research and preventive measures, enhancing their ability to make informed decisions about their health.

In addition to professional support, connecting with community resources can play a significant role in risk reduction. Local organizations often provide valuable information about esophageal cancer, including educational workshops, support groups, and resources for healthy living. Engaging with these community initiatives not only provides access to essential information but also fosters a sense of belonging and shared purpose.

Finding like-minded individuals who are also focused on reducing their risk can create a motivating atmosphere where members can exchange tips, experiences, and encouragement. Family and friends form the cornerstone of an effective support system. It is vital for individuals to communicate their concerns about esophageal cancer and their desire to adopt healthier lifestyles.

By sharing their goals with loved ones, individuals can enlist their support in making dietary changes, engaging in regular physical activity, or avoiding harmful habits such as smoking and excessive alcohol consumption.

This communal effort can strengthen relationships and create a network of accountability, where friends and family members encourage each other to stick to their health goals.

Online platforms and social media can also serve as valuable tools for building a support system. Virtual communities dedicated to health and wellness provide access to a wealth of information and allow individuals to connect with others facing similar challenges. Online forums and social media groups can facilitate discussions on esophageal cancer prevention, share success stories, and provide emotional support. By participating in these digital communities, individuals can find inspiration and motivation, further enhancing their commitment to reducing their risk of esophageal cancer.

In conclusion, building a support system is an integral part of a comprehensive strategy for reducing the risk of esophageal cancer. By connecting with healthcare professionals, engaging with community resources, relying on the support of family and friends, and utilizing online platforms, individuals can create a strong network that empowers them to make informed choices about their health. This collaborative approach not only enhances knowledge and motivation but also fosters resilience in the face of health challenges, ultimately contributing to more effective risk reduction efforts.

# How To Reduce Esophageal Cancer Risk

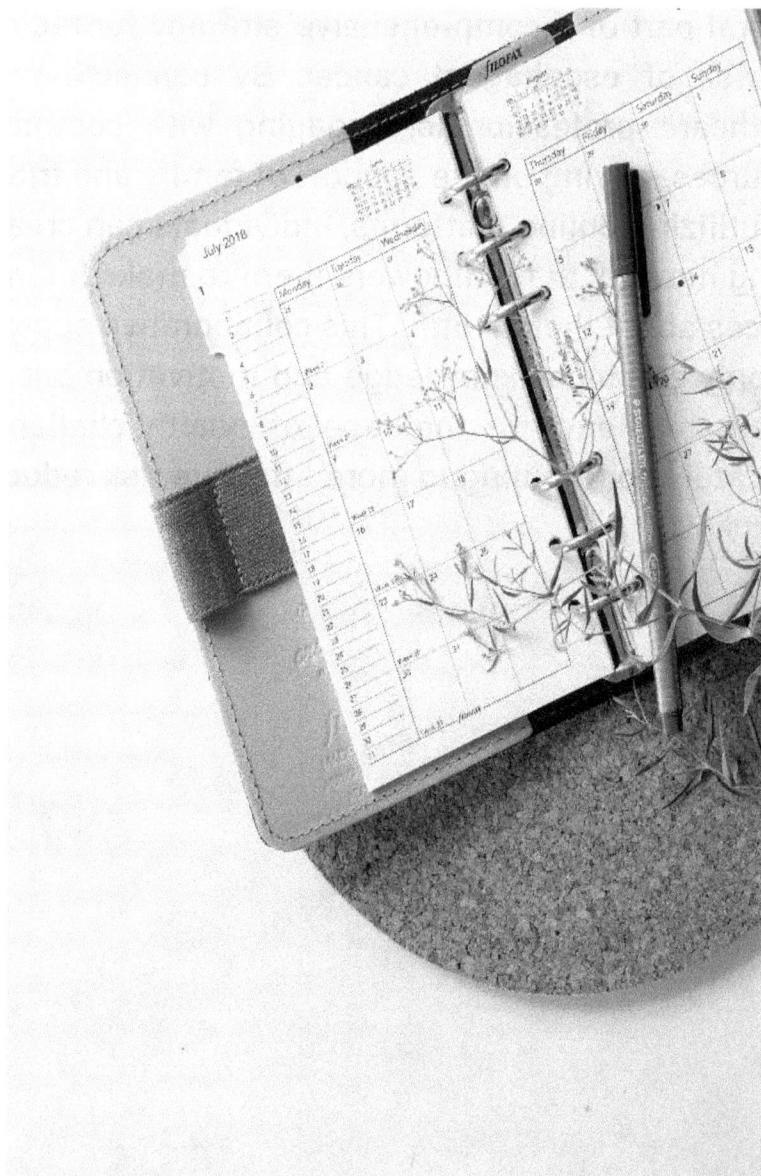

# Chapter 10

# Taking Action: Creating Your Personalized Risk Reduction Plan

## Assessing Your Current Risks

Assessing your current risks is a crucial first step in taking proactive measures to reduce the likelihood of developing esophageal cancer. Understanding the factors that contribute to your personal risk profile can empower you to make informed decisions about your health. This process involves evaluating both genetic and lifestyle factors that may elevate your risk, as well as understanding the symptoms and signs that could indicate an underlying issue.

Genetic predisposition plays a significant role in assessing your risk for esophageal cancer. Individuals with a family history of the disease, particularly those with relatives who have had esophageal or other related cancers, should consider genetic counseling and testing.

Additionally, certain genetic syndromes, such as Barrett's esophagus or Lynch syndrome, can predispose individuals to esophageal cancer. Gaining awareness of these hereditary factors can help you and your healthcare provider determine a tailored surveillance and prevention strategy.

Lifestyle choices significantly impact your overall risk for esophageal cancer. Factors such as smoking, excessive alcohol consumption, and obesity are well-documented contributors to the disease. For example, smoking introduces harmful carcinogens into the body, while alcohol can irritate the esophagus and promote the development of precancerous conditions. Evaluating your own habits and making adjustments—such as quitting smoking, moderating alcohol intake, and maintaining a healthy weight—can substantially lower your risk.

Dietary considerations also play an essential role in assessing your risk. Consuming a diet rich in fruits, vegetables, and whole grains while limiting processed foods and red meats can help mitigate the risk of esophageal cancer.

Certain dietary components, like antioxidants and fiber, have been linked to a reduced risk of various cancers, including esophageal. Keeping a food diary can help you reflect on your eating patterns and identify areas for improvement, making it easier to implement healthier choices.

Finally, regular medical check-ups and screenings are vital in assessing your risk for esophageal cancer. If you experience symptoms such as persistent heartburn, difficulty swallowing, or unexplained weight loss, it is important to consult a healthcare professional for further evaluation.

Early detection is key in managing health conditions effectively, and your doctor may recommend specific tests or referrals to specialists based on your risk factors. By actively assessing your current risks, you can take significant strides toward reducing your chances of developing esophageal cancer and enhancing your overall well-being.

## Setting Realistic Goals

Setting realistic goals is a crucial component of any strategy aimed at reducing the risk of esophageal cancer. While it may be tempting to adopt sweeping changes in lifestyle or diet, establishing practical, attainable objectives can lead to more sustainable habits over time.

This subchapter will explore how to effectively set these goals and incorporate them into daily life, ultimately fostering a proactive approach to health that can significantly mitigate cancer risk.

The first step in setting realistic goals is to perform a thorough assessment of current habits and health status. Understanding personal risk factors, such as family history, dietary choices, lifestyle practices, and existing health issues, provides a baseline from which to draw. Individuals should consider keeping a journal or using an app to track their eating habits, exercise routines, and any symptoms they may experience.

This self-reflection not only highlights areas for improvement but also enables individuals to set specific, measurable goals that are tailored to their unique circumstances.

Next, it is essential to break larger health objectives into smaller, manageable tasks. For instance, if the goal is to increase fruit and vegetable intake, individuals might start by committing to include one additional serving of vegetables in their meals each day. Gradually increasing this target over time can lead to a more significant dietary shift without feeling overwhelming. This incremental approach is effective in cultivating long-lasting habits and reducing the likelihood of burnout or discouragement that can arise from overly ambitious goals.

Additionally, it is important to remain flexible and adaptable when pursuing these goals. Life circumstances often change, and so might the feasibility of certain objectives. For example, if a busy work schedule prevents regular meal prep, individuals might adjust their goal to include healthier options when dining out or utilizing ready-to-eat, nutritious foods.

Being open to modifying goals ensures that they remain realistic and achievable, allowing individuals to stay on track even when faced with unexpected challenges.

Lastly, seeking support from friends, family, or healthcare professionals can enhance goal-setting efforts significantly. Sharing objectives with others creates accountability and can lead to a community of encouragement. Whether it's joining a local support group focused on health and wellness or engaging with a nutritionist for personalized guidance, collaboration can provide valuable resources and motivation.

Setting realistic goals in this manner not only empowers individuals to take control of their health but also fosters a sense of shared commitment to reducing esophageal cancer risk within their communities.

## Tracking Progress and Adjustments

Tracking progress and making adjustments are critical components in the journey of reducing esophageal cancer risk. For individuals concerned about their health, understanding how to effectively monitor their efforts can lead to more significant outcomes. This subchapter will outline practical methods for tracking progress, the importance of regular evaluations, and strategies for making necessary adjustments to ensure continued risk reduction.

One effective method of tracking progress is through the establishment of specific, measurable goals. Individuals should start by assessing their current habits related to diet, lifestyle, and medical check-ups. For example, setting a goal to increase the intake of fruits and vegetables can be measured by daily servings. Likewise, monitoring weight changes, smoking cessation, or alcohol consumption can provide clear indicators of progress.

Keeping a journal or using mobile applications to log these metrics can serve as a visual reminder of one's efforts and accomplishments, fostering a sense of accountability.

Regular self-assessment is also essential for understanding how well one is doing in risk reduction efforts. Monthly reviews of health habits can help identify trends, revealing whether certain strategies are effective or if they need to be adjusted. For instance, if an individual notices a recurring pattern of heartburn or acid reflux despite dietary changes, it may indicate the need for further medical evaluation or lifestyle modifications. Seeking feedback from healthcare professionals during routine check-ups can provide additional insights and help individuals stay on track with their goals.

In conjunction with monitoring progress, it is vital to remain adaptable in one's approach. The body's responses to dietary changes, exercise, and other lifestyle adjustments can vary significantly from person to person. Therefore, what works for one individual may not yield the same results for another.

If certain strategies seem ineffective, it is crucial to reassess and consider alternative approaches, such as consulting with a nutritionist or participating in support groups. This flexibility not only enhances the likelihood of success but also reinforces the importance of a personalized risk reduction plan.

Finally, celebrating milestones along the way can help maintain motivation and commitment to reducing esophageal cancer risk. Recognizing achievements, no matter how small, can provide encouragement and a sense of accomplishment. Whether it's reaching a weight goal, achieving a certain number of smoke-free days, or simply feeling better overall, acknowledging these victories can bolster the resolve to continue making healthy choices.

Additionally, sharing successes with friends or family can create a supportive network that reinforces positive behaviors and fosters a community dedicated to health.

In conclusion, tracking progress and making adjustments are integral to the ongoing process of reducing esophageal cancer risk. By setting measurable goals, conducting regular self-assessments, remaining adaptable, and celebrating achievements, individuals can create a robust framework for their health journey. This proactive approach not only empowers individuals but also enhances their understanding of the steps necessary to mitigate their risk of esophageal cancer effectively.

# How To Reduce Esophageal Cancer Risk

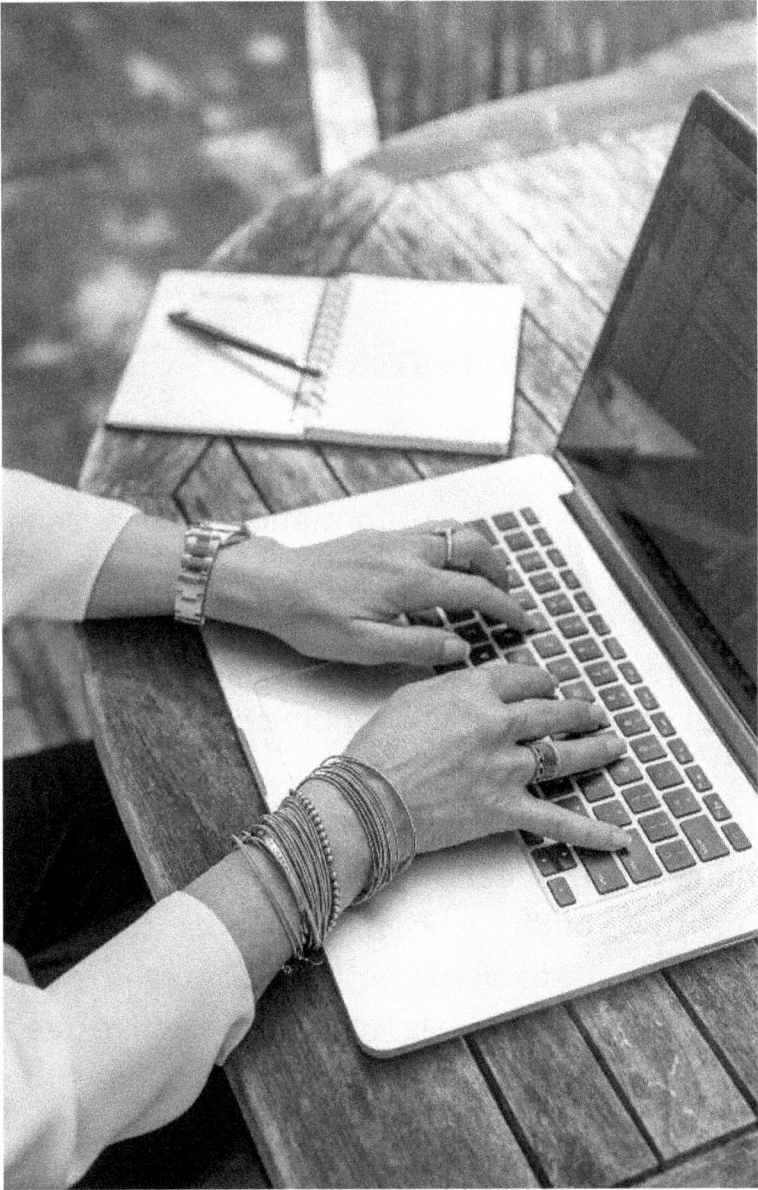

# Chapter 11

# Resources for Further Support

## Organizations and Support Groups

Organizations and support groups play a vital role in providing resources, information, and a sense of community for individuals concerned about esophageal cancer. These entities are dedicated to raising awareness, funding research, and offering practical strategies for risk reduction.

By connecting with these organizations, individuals can access reliable information and find support from others who share similar concerns and experiences. Understanding the resources available can empower individuals to take proactive steps in reducing their risk of esophageal cancer.

One of the primary organizations focused on esophageal cancer is the Esophageal Cancer Awareness Association (ECAA). This nonprofit organization is committed to increasing awareness of esophageal cancer and its risk factors. Through educational programs, community outreach, and advocacy efforts, the ECAA provides valuable information about lifestyle changes that can help lower the risk of developing this cancer.

Their website offers a wealth of resources, including guidelines on diet, smoking cessation, and the importance of regular medical check-ups, which are crucial for early detection and prevention.

Another significant organization is the American Cancer Society (ACS), which offers comprehensive information on various types of cancer, including esophageal cancer. The ACS emphasizes the importance of a healthy lifestyle as a means of reducing cancer risk. Their resources cover a wide range of topics, from nutritional guidelines to the benefits of physical activity.

They also provide information about the role of screening and surveillance in detecting esophageal cancer early, which can greatly improve outcomes. By participating in ACS-sponsored events or utilizing their online resources, individuals can stay informed about the latest research and recommendations for reducing risk.

Support groups also play a crucial role in the journey of individuals concerned about esophageal cancer. These groups provide a platform for sharing experiences, fears, and strategies related to cancer prevention and health maintenance. Connecting with others who understand the challenges can help alleviate feelings of isolation and anxiety.

Many organizations, such as the ECAA and ACS, offer online forums and local meetings where individuals can discuss their concerns and learn from one another. This communal aspect often fosters motivation and accountability, encouraging participants to adopt healthier lifestyles collectively.

In addition to providing emotional support, many organizations offer educational workshops and seminars focused on risk reduction strategies. These events often feature experts in nutrition, exercise, and oncology who provide insights on evidence-based practices for reducing esophageal cancer risk. Attending these workshops allows individuals to ask questions, engage with professionals, and gain practical knowledge that can be applied to their daily lives.

By actively participating in these educational opportunities, individuals can enhance their understanding of esophageal cancer and implement effective risk-reduction strategies.

Engaging with organizations and support groups dedicated to esophageal cancer not only enhances individual knowledge and skills but also fosters a sense of community and collective action. As individuals work together to share resources and experiences, they create a supportive environment that promotes healthy living and cancer prevention.

By leveraging these resources, individuals concerned about esophageal cancer can take significant steps toward reducing their risk and improving their overall health.

## Educational Materials and Websites

Educational materials and websites play a crucial role in empowering individuals concerned about esophageal cancer. Knowledge is a powerful tool for prevention, and a wealth of resources is available to help people understand their risk factors and the steps they can take to reduce them.

From brochures and pamphlets to online platforms, these materials provide essential information on esophageal cancer, its causes, and strategies for maintaining esophageal health. They often include guidelines on diet, lifestyle changes, and regular screenings, which are pivotal in minimizing risk.

Prominent health organizations, such as the American Cancer Society and the National Cancer Institute, offer extensive resources dedicated to esophageal cancer. Their websites feature sections specifically focused on prevention and risk reduction. These platforms provide evidence-based information on the importance of maintaining a healthy weight, avoiding tobacco, and moderating alcohol consumption.

Furthermore, they often share the latest research findings, which can help individuals stay informed about emerging risk factors and innovative prevention strategies.

In addition to national health organizations, local cancer centers and hospitals produce educational materials tailored to their communities. These resources often include information on local support groups, screening programs, and workshops that emphasize healthy lifestyle choices.

By connecting individuals with local resources, these institutions foster a supportive environment where people can learn and share experiences related to esophageal cancer prevention. This localized approach can enhance the effectiveness of education by making it more relatable and accessible.

Online courses and webinars are increasingly popular as educational tools for those concerned about esophageal cancer. These digital platforms provide flexible learning opportunities, allowing participants to engage with experts in the field from the comfort of their homes.

Topics covered may include the role of diet in cancer prevention, the impact of reflux disease, and the importance of early detection. Interactive formats can stimulate discussion and allow individuals to ask questions directly, fostering a deeper understanding of risk reduction strategies.

Finally, social media platforms and online support groups have emerged as vital resources for individuals seeking community and information. These spaces allow for the sharing of personal stories and experiences, which can be incredibly valuable for those grappling with the fear of esophageal cancer. Many organizations utilize social media to disseminate educational content, promote awareness campaigns, and connect individuals with similar concerns. By leveraging these digital resources, individuals can gain insights into practical strategies for reducing their risk while finding a sense of camaraderie and support in their journey toward better esophageal health.

## Professional Guidance and Counseling Options

Professional guidance and counseling play a crucial role in the proactive management of health risks, including esophageal cancer. Individuals who are concerned about their risk of developing this type of cancer can benefit significantly from engaging with healthcare professionals who specialize in cancer prevention and risk assessment.

These professionals offer tailored strategies designed to educate patients about their risk factors, recommend appropriate screenings, and provide guidance on lifestyle modifications that can mitigate those risks. Consulting with a healthcare provider can help individuals identify personal risk factors, such as genetic predispositions or existing medical conditions, and develop a customized plan to reduce their likelihood of developing esophageal cancer.

One of the primary avenues for professional guidance is through genetic counseling. For those with a family history of esophageal cancer or related conditions, genetic counselors can offer insights into hereditary cancer syndromes and the implications for personal health. This type of counseling includes assessing family medical histories, discussing the potential need for genetic testing, and interpreting test results. Understanding one's genetic makeup can empower individuals to make informed decisions about their health, including the adoption of more rigorous screening protocols or preventive measures.

In addition to genetic counseling, dietary and nutritional counseling can provide significant benefits. Nutritionists and dietitians can help individuals identify foods that may increase their risk of esophageal cancer, such as those high in processed sugars or unhealthy fats. They can also promote a diet rich in fruits, vegetables, whole grains, and lean proteins, which are known to have protective effects against cancer.

By working with a nutrition professional, individuals can create meal plans that not only support overall health but also specifically target risk reduction for esophageal cancer.

Mental health support is another essential aspect of professional guidance in risk reduction. The emotional toll of worrying about cancer can lead to anxiety, depression, and unhealthy coping mechanisms, which may inadvertently increase risk factors for esophageal cancer, such as smoking or excessive alcohol consumption.

Professional counselors and therapists can offer strategies to manage stress and anxiety, helping individuals develop healthier coping skills. Furthermore, support groups can provide a sense of community, allowing individuals to share their concerns and experiences while learning from others facing similar challenges.

Finally, healthcare professionals can keep patients informed about the latest research and advancements in esophageal cancer prevention. Regular consultations with oncologists or specialists in preventive medicine can ensure that individuals receive updated information on emerging risk factors, new screening methods, and innovative lifestyle strategies. This ongoing engagement with healthcare providers can foster a proactive approach to health management, enabling individuals to take charge of their well-being and significantly reduce their risk of esophageal cancer. By leveraging professional guidance and counseling options, individuals can build a robust support network that empowers them on their journey toward better health.

# How To Reduce Esophageal Cancer Risk

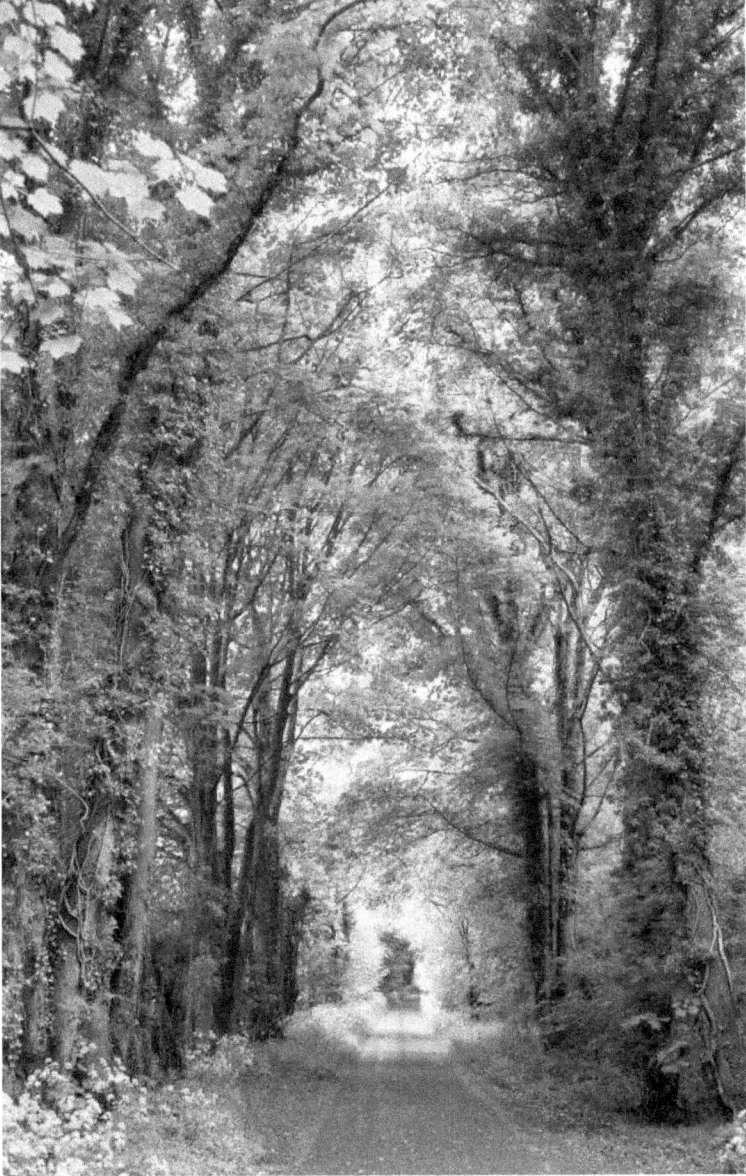

# Chapter 12

# Conclusion: Empowering Yourself Against Esophageal Cancer

## Recap of Key Strategies

In the pursuit of reducing the risk of esophageal cancer, it is essential to recap the key strategies that have emerged from the latest research and expert recommendations. This subchapter aims to distill these strategies into actionable steps for individuals concerned about their health. By understanding these strategies, readers can take proactive measures to enhance their well-being and mitigate the potential risks associated with esophageal cancer.

One of the primary strategies for reducing esophageal cancer risk is to maintain a healthy weight. Obesity has been identified as a significant risk factor for this type of cancer, particularly due to its association with gastroesophageal reflux disease (GERD).

Individuals should aim for a balanced diet rich in fruits, vegetables, whole grains, and lean proteins while minimizing processed foods, sugars, and unhealthy fats. Regular physical activity is equally important; engaging in at least 150 minutes of moderate aerobic exercise per week can help individuals achieve and maintain a healthy weight, thereby lowering their risk.

Another critical strategy involves dietary modifications that focus on reducing acid reflux and promoting overall digestive health. Avoiding trigger foods such as spicy dishes, citrus fruits, and high-fat meals can significantly decrease the likelihood of GERD, which is linked to esophageal cancer.

Additionally, incorporating foods high in antioxidants, such as berries, nuts, and green leafy vegetables, can support cellular health and may help protect against cancerous changes in the esophagus. It is also advisable to eat smaller, more frequent meals and to refrain from lying down immediately after eating.

Quitting smoking and limiting alcohol consumption are vital components of a comprehensive risk reduction plan. Tobacco use is a well-established risk factor for several types of cancer, including esophageal cancer. For those who smoke, seeking resources to quit can have immediate and long-term health benefits. Similarly, limiting alcohol intake to moderate levels—defined as up to one drink per day for women and two for men—can further decrease the risk. Understanding the cumulative effect of these lifestyle choices is crucial in fostering an environment conducive to health.

Regular medical check-ups and screenings also play a significant role in risk reduction. Individuals with risk factors such as chronic GERD or a family history of esophageal cancer should discuss the possibility of endoscopic screenings with their healthcare provider. Early detection of precancerous conditions, such as Barrett's esophagus, can lead to timely interventions and significantly improve outcomes. Staying informed about personal health and any symptoms that could indicate an issue is paramount for proactive management.

In summary, reducing the risk of esophageal cancer involves a multi-faceted approach that encompasses healthy weight management, dietary adjustments, lifestyle changes, and regular health screenings. Emphasizing a holistic strategy empowers individuals to take control of their health and make informed choices that can lead to a significant reduction in their risk. As awareness grows and these strategies are embraced, individuals can foster a healthier future, contributing to the overall decline in esophageal cancer incidence.

## The Importance of Staying Informed

Staying informed is a fundamental aspect of effective risk reduction, particularly when it comes to esophageal cancer. Knowledge equips individuals with the tools to make informed decisions about their health and lifestyle choices. This subchapter will explore the significance of being well-informed about esophageal cancer, including its risk factors, symptoms, and prevention strategies.

As individuals become more aware of the nuances associated with esophageal cancer, they can take proactive steps to mitigate their risk and improve their overall well-being.

Understanding the risk factors associated with esophageal cancer is crucial for anyone concerned about their health. Esophageal cancer can be influenced by various elements, including lifestyle choices, dietary habits, and underlying health conditions. For instance, smoking and excessive alcohol consumption have been consistently linked to a higher risk of developing this type of cancer.

Additionally, chronic acid reflux, or gastroesophageal reflux disease (GERD), can lead to Barrett's esophagus, a condition that significantly increases the risk of esophageal cancer. By staying informed about these risk factors, individuals can make conscious choices to reduce their exposure and, in turn, their risk.

Recognizing the early symptoms of esophageal cancer is equally important. Symptoms such as difficulty swallowing, persistent heartburn, unexplained weight loss, and chest pain may indicate a problem that warrants further investigation. Early detection of esophageal cancer can greatly improve treatment outcomes, making it essential for individuals to be vigilant about any changes in their health.

Staying informed about these warning signs allows individuals to seek medical advice promptly, facilitating early diagnosis and intervention, which are critical in effectively managing the disease.

Moreover, knowledge about preventive measures can empower individuals to take control of their health. This includes adopting a balanced diet rich in fruits, vegetables, and whole grains while limiting processed foods, red meats, and sugars. Regular physical activity, maintaining a healthy weight, and avoiding tobacco products are also vital components of a lifestyle that can help reduce the risk of esophageal cancer.

By integrating these strategies into daily life, individuals can significantly lower their risk and foster a healthier lifestyle. Staying informed about these practical strategies enables individuals to make informed choices that align with their health goals.

Lastly, utilizing credible resources and support networks can enhance one's ability to stay informed. Engaging with healthcare professionals, participating in community health programs, and accessing reputable online resources can provide valuable insights into esophageal cancer prevention. Furthermore, connecting with support groups can offer emotional backing and shared experiences, which can be beneficial for individuals navigating their health concerns.

By fostering a culture of continuous learning and openness to information, individuals can cultivate a proactive approach to their health, ultimately reducing their risk of esophageal cancer and enhancing their quality of life.

## Encouragement for Ongoing Prevention Efforts

In the journey toward reducing the risk of esophageal cancer, sustained encouragement for ongoing prevention efforts is vital. Individuals concerned about their health need to understand that the fight against cancer is a continuous process that involves proactive lifestyle choices and regular monitoring.

Establishing a solid foundation of knowledge about risk factors and preventive measures can empower individuals to take charge of their health and make informed decisions that significantly lower their risk of developing this serious condition.

One of the most effective strategies for reducing esophageal cancer risk is maintaining a healthy diet. Research has shown that a diet rich in fruits, vegetables, whole grains, and lean proteins can have a protective effect against various types of cancer, including esophageal cancer.

Antioxidants found in colorful fruits and vegetables, like berries and leafy greens, can combat oxidative stress, while whole grains provide essential nutrients and fiber that support digestive health. Encouraging individuals to incorporate these foods into their daily meals can foster a long-term commitment to healthier eating habits.

In addition to dietary changes, promoting regular physical activity plays a crucial role in cancer prevention. Engaging in consistent exercise not only helps maintain a healthy weight but also reduces the risk of conditions such as gastroesophageal reflux disease (GERD), a significant risk factor for esophageal cancer.

Encouragement to find enjoyable forms of exercise, whether through walking, swimming, or group classes, can motivate individuals to integrate physical activity into their routines. This approach not only improves physical health but also enhances mental well-being, creating a holistic focus on prevention.

Quitting smoking and moderating alcohol intake are other essential components of an effective risk reduction strategy. Smoking is a well-documented risk factor for esophageal cancer, and cessation programs can provide the necessary support for individuals looking to quit.

Similarly, educating individuals about the risks associated with excessive alcohol consumption and promoting moderation can lead to significant health benefits. Encouragement and resources for smoking cessation and responsible drinking can foster a supportive community where individuals feel empowered to make these critical lifestyle changes.

Finally, ongoing education and regular health screenings are fundamental in the fight against esophageal cancer. Individuals should be encouraged to stay informed about the latest research and advancements in cancer prevention and detection. Regular check-ups with healthcare providers can help identify any potential issues early on, allowing for timely intervention.

By cultivating a culture of awareness and proactive health management, individuals can feel confident in their ability to reduce their risk of esophageal cancer, turning their concerns into actionable steps for a healthier future.

# Author Notes & Acknowledgments

First and foremost, I would like to express my deepest gratitude to the people who inspired and supported me throughout the journey of writing this book. This project would not have been possible without their unwavering belief in me and their invaluable contributions.

To my wife, thank you for your constant encouragement and understanding. Your love and support have been my anchor during the challenging times of researching and writing this book. Your belief in my ability to make a difference in people's lives has been my driving force.

I would also like to disclose that this book contains some renewed artificial intelligence-generated content. I really appreciate very recent technological innovation by outstanding scientists and of course our reader's understanding.

Lastly, I want to express my deepest gratitude to the readers of this book. I sincerely hope the strategies and methods outlined within these pages will provide you with the knowledge and tools needed to truly make your life much better. Your commitment to seeking any good solutions and willingness to explore multiple methods is commendable.

# Author Bio

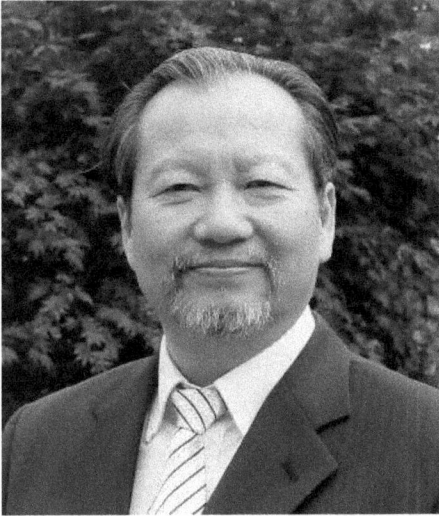

Johnson Wu earned his MD in 1982. With over 40 years of clinical experience, he has worked in hospitals in Zhejiang and Shanghai, China, as well as the Royal Marsden Hospital (part of Imperial College) in London, UK.

Upon the recommendation of Sir Aaron Klug, the president of The Royal Society and a Nobel Prize winner in Chemistry, Dr. Wu was honorably awarded a British Royal Society Fellowship. He has published medical books and articles in seven countries and currently practices medicine in Canada.

www.ingramcontent.com/pod-product-compliance
Lightning Source LLC
Chambersburg PA
CBHW060236030426
42335CB00014B/1491